WHITE BLOOD CELLS

MICROCIRCULATION REVIEWS 1

H. SCHMID-SCHÖNBEIN and G.W. SCHMID-SCHÖNBEIN, Series Editors

WHITE BLOOD CELLS

MORPHOLOGY AND RHEOLOGY AS RELATED TO FUNCTION

Proceedings, with Commentary, of the Symposium held at London, England
October 3–4, 1981

edited by

U. BAGGE
Laboratory of Experimental Biology
Dept. of Anatomy
University of Göteborg
Göteborg
Sweden

G.V.R. BORN
Dept. of Pharmacology
University of London
King's College
Strand
London
United Kingdom

P. GAEHTGENS
Institut für Normale und Pathologische Physiologie
Universität zu Köln
Köln
Germany

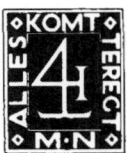

SPRINGER-SCIENCE+BUSINESS MEDIA, B.V.

Distributors:

for the United States and Canada
Kluwer Boston, Inc.
190 Old Derby Street
Hingham, MA 02043
USA

for all other countries
Kluwer Academic Publishers Group
Distribution Center
P.O.Box 322
3300 AH Dordrecht
The Netherlands

Library of Congress Cataloging in Publication Data
Main entry under title:

White blood cells.

   (Microcirculation reviews ; v. 1)
   1. Leucocytes--Congresses. 2. Rheology
(Biology)--Congresses. I. Bagge, U. II. Born, –
G. V. R. III. Gaehtgens, P. IV. Series. [DNLM:
1. Leukocytes--Physiology--Congresses. 2. Blood
flow velocity--Congresses. W1 MI298M v. 1 / WH
200 W582 1981]
QP95.W44   612'.112   82-7117
                  AACR2

ISBN 978-94-009-7587-3   ISBN 978-94-009-7585-9 (eBook)
DOI 10.1007/978-94-009-7585-9

CONTENTS

VI

CONTENTS,continued

LIST of PARTICIPANTS

J.P.ABITA, Service de Médecine Nucléaire Pr. Najean, Hopital
Saint-Louis,2 Place du Dr. Fournier,75474 Paris Cedex 1o, France

B.AMUNDSON, Laboratory of Exp. Biology, Dept. of Anatomy,
University of Göteborg, Box 33o31, S-4oo33 Göteborg, Sweden

U.BAGGE, Laboratory of Exp. Biology, Dept. of Anatomy,
University of Göteborg, Box 33o31, S-4oo33 Göteborg, Sweden

P.-I.BRANEMARK, Laboratory of Exp. Biology, Dept. of Anatomy
University of Göteborg, Box 33o31, S-4oo33 Göteborg, Sweden

G.V.R.BORN, Dept. of Pharmacology, University of London,
King's College, Strand, London WC 2R 2LS, U.K.

S.CHIEN, Dept. of Physiology, Columbia University, College of
Physicians and Surgeons, 63o West 168th St., New York,
N.Y. 1oo32, USA

G.R.COKELET, Dept. of Radiation Biology and Biophysics,University
of Rochester,Med. Center,6o1 Elmwood Ave, Rochester,N.Y.14642,USA

J.FEHR, Abteilung für Hämatologie, Medizinische Klinik CH 5
Universitätsspital, CH-8o91 Zürich, Switzerland

P. GAEHTGENS, Institut für Normale und Pathologische Physiologie,
Universität zu Köln, Robert-Koch-Str. 39, 5ooo Köln 41, Germany

G.HOPEN, Medical Dept. B, University of Bergen, Haukeland
sykehus, N-5o16 Bergen, Norway

P.LaCELLE,Dept. of Radiation Biology and Biophysics, University of
Rochester, Med. Center, 6o1 Elmwood Ave, Rochester, N.Y.14642, USA

J.M.LACKIE, Dept. of Cell Biology, Glasgow University,
Glasgow G12 8QQ, U.K.

M.LICHTMAN, Dept.of Medicine, University of Rochester, School
of Medicine, 6o1 Elmwood Ave, Rochester, N.Y. 14642, USA

P.C.MALONE, Dept. of Exp. Pathology, University of Birmingham,
273 Kingsbury Rd., Erdington, Birmingham B24 8RD, U.K.

H.N.MAYROVITZ, Miami Heart Institute, 47o1 N. Meridean Ave,
Miami Beach, Florida 33322, USA

R.R.McGREGOR, Infectious Diseases Section, 536 Johnson Pavilion/
G2, University of Pennsylvania, School of Medicine, Philadelphia,
Pa. 191o4, USA

U.NOBIS,Institut für Normale und Pathologische Physiologie,
Universität zu Köln, Robert-Koch-Str. 39, 5ooo Köln 41, Germany

D.M.V. PARROTT, Bacteriology and Immunology Dept., University
of Glasgow (Western Infirmary), Glasgow G11 6NT, U.K.

J.D.PEARSON, A.R.C. Institute of Animal Physiology, Babraham,
Cambridge CB2 4AT, U.K.

G.W.SCHMID-SCHÖNBEIN, Dept. of Appl. Mechanics and Eng.Sciences,
Bioengineering, UCSD, La Jolla, Cal. 92o93, USA

R.SKALAK, Bioengineering Institute, Dept. of Civil Engineering
and Eng. Mechanics, Columbia University, New York, N.Y.1oo27, USA

L.H.SMAJE,Dept. of Physiology, Charing Cross Hosp.Medical School,
Fulham Palace Road, London W6 8RF, U.K.

J.L.WAUTIER, Dept. Immunohematology, Hopital Lariboisière,
2 Rue A. Paré, 75475 Paris Cedex 1o, France

M.P.WIEDEMAN, Dept. of Physiology, Temple Medical School,
Philadelphia, Pa. 1914o, USA

P.C.WILKINSON, Bacteriology and Immunology Dept., University of
Glasgow (Western Infirmary), Glasgow G11 6NT, U.K.

T.J.WILLIAMS, Dept. of Pharmac., Royal College of Surgeons of
England, 35/43 Lincoln's Inn Fields, London, WC2A 3PN, U.K.

PREFACE:

HOW COULD WHITE BLOOD CELL RHEOLOGY BE RELATED TO WHITE BLOOD CELL FUNCTION?

Following delivery from the production sites into the peripheral blood, the life span of an "average WBC" may somewhat arbitrarily be divided into an inactive phase, during which the cell is passively transported by the circulation, and an active phase, during which it moves through the vascular wall and into the tissue spaces where its physiological function is fulfilled. Various and complex phenomena contribute to the behaviour of WBCs in these two phases of their life, some of which are governed by the cell's own physical properties and by alterations of these properties brought about in response to external stimuli. The events constituting the transition between these phases seem to be of particular interest. While many of the biochemical aspects of these events have attracted considerable attention in the past, the present workshop was primarily focussed at the biophysical properties of WBCs and their alterations during their life span, in accordance with the general topic "WBC RHEOLOGY AS RELATED TO FUNCTION".

The physiological function of WBCs is related to that of the microcirculation, if one accepts the latter to be directed towards the distribution of materials exchanged between the intra- and extravascular space. Conversely, microcirculatory function may appear related to WBC function, if the response of the terminal vasculature to local stimuli, e.g. under conditions of inflammation, is considered. Despite this functional interrelationship the flow properties and the flow behaviour of normal WBCs in the smallest blood vessels have not received much attention from microcirculatory researchers, in part as a result of methodical difficulties. It is certainly due to the relatively low concentration of WBC in the circulating blood that by far more efforts have been made to study red blood cell behaviour.

The diameter of nutritive capillaries, e.g. in the myocardium or in skeletal muscle, is substantially less than that of the red cells and certainly of the WBCs. How is it possible that the presence of the rather unpliable WBCs does not interfere with the subtle balance between local blood supply and local metabolic demand, which is so characteristic of the normal microcirculation? How can capillary circulation be maintained under conditions of disease associated with increased WBC concentration in the blood? Rough calculation on the basis of deformation times shows that at elevated WBC concentration of, say $20 \cdot 10^3$/ul a capillary of 5um diameter could be shut off from active perfusion during 50% of total time. This means that during leukocytosis approximately 50% of all myocardial and skeletal muscle capillaries would be occluded by slowly deforming WBCs. It may thus seem conceivable that the necessity of providing a large number of WBC to a tissue area inflicted in an inflammatory reaction may also be associated with a significant interference with capillary circulation in this area.

Another aspect of the relationship between WBC rheology and microcirculatory flow is the problem of margination. It seems well established that emigration of activated leukocytes occurs only from post-capillary venules. Although the close proximity between the WBC membrane surface and the endothelium in the smallest capillaries may render these vessels ideal sites for emigration, the WBCs do not seem to take advantage of this "topographical benefit". In contrast, they prefer emigration from venules, which, however, requires that they must establish contact with th venular wall before being able to adhere and penetrate. Even if activated, the leukocyte would not be able to make its way into the interstitium unless it is passively transported towards the endothelial lining of the postcapillary venules. How does the WBC get to the vessel wall? Is this a consequence of its own behaviou in flow? How is the probability of establishing contact with the vessel wall affected by changes in blood flow?

It is quite obvious that WBC rheology is of particular relevance in conjunction with active locomotion of these cells through endothelium and tissue spaces. Margination, adhesion, and locomotion can be regarded as different (although interrelated) phenomena in which mechanical and biochemical factors may be of equal importance. The mechanism of locomotion requires continuous establishment and de-establishment of intimate contact between the cell surface and that of the substratum, but it also requires the controlled initiation of intracellular mechanisms converting the relatively rigid non-active WBC into a fluid body which continuously undergoes shape changes.

Finally, the emigration of WBCs requires the existence of preformed "holes" or the formation of such passageways by some WBC endothelium interaction of unknown nature. Why is the site of this phenomenon limited to post-capillary venules, and what are the consequences of WBC passage through the endothelium for the barrier function of the vascular wall?

It was the purpose of this workshop to stimulate discussion on these various aspects between representatives of scientific disciplines who otherwise might not have been in contact. The main idea therefore was one of "interdisciplinary cross-fertilization" (BRANEMARK). This volume contains the presentations of the contributors and interspersed commentaries, which serve to summarize both the commentators views and the discussion at the workshop. Organizers and participants owe special gratitude to the CIBA FOUNDATION (41 Portland Place, London, U.K.) who generously supported the meeting by providing an environment which could not have been more suitable for an informal and effervescent exchange of knowledge and ideas. Fertilization in the literal sense requires a fertilizer and the soil to be fertilized - but no crop will be harvested unless sun and rain have contributed to its growth.

U. Bagge

G.V.R. Born

P. Gaehtgens

ANALYSIS OF WHITE BLOOD CELL DEFORMATION

R. SKALAK , G.W. SCHMID-SCHÖNBEIN , S. CHIEN

1. INTRODUCTION

In vivo observations in man (1) indicate that compared
to red blood cells the leukocyte is relatively stiff and
deforms more slowly. Experiments on the flow of leukocytes
through tapering glass capillaries (2) and by the use of
micropipettes (3,4) quantitatively confirm the impression
that white cells deform slowly under a constant stress field.
These observations require that any model of the white cell
contain a viscous element. Experiments in tapered capillaries
(2) and in micropipettes (4) indicate that if a stress is
suddenly applied to a white blood cell, it responds with some
deformation very rapidly and then continues its slow deformation. These characteristics require that any model also
contain an elastic element in series with the viscous element.
A model consisting of an elastic element and a fluid element
in series is the so-called Maxwell model. Such a model, if
deformed and held in a fixed position for sufficient time,
would not recover its shape upon release of the stress. But
observations after the release of stress in tapered capillaries
(2) and micropipettes experiments (4) show that the white cell
after deformation, will recover its spherical shape in a few
seconds or longer. This indicates that a parallel elastic
element must be provided in order to restore the cell to its
original shape.

The simplest model that can meet all the requirements is
a three element viscoelastic material shown schematically
in Fig. 1. This model is rheologically equivalent to the
standard solid model shown in Fig. 2. The elastic coefficients

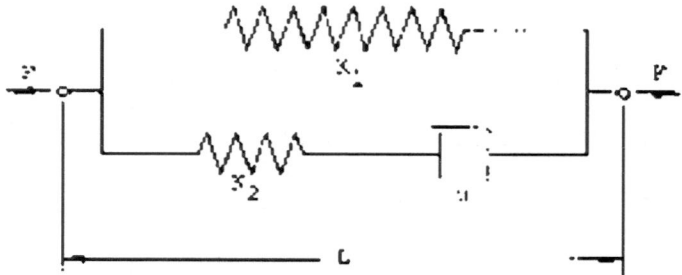

FIGURE 1. Three element model used to represent white blood cell cytoplasm (4) or the cell as a whole (2). The model shown is a Maxwell fluid (K_2, μ) in parallel with a restoring spring (K_1).

of the springs in Fig. 1, K_1, K_2 are not equal to the spring constants K_1', K_2' in Fig. 2, but the two sets of spring constants can be related. The model shown in Fig. 1 is pre-ferred to represent the white blood cell because the spring constant K_1 in this case represents the weak restoring force which eventually returns the cell to its original shape with no stress present. This elasticity may be due to the cyto-plasm itself, or to membrane and surface forces. It is also possible that the Brownian motion of the granules and cyto-plasm of the cell play a role in the gradual restoration of spherical shape of the cell. The membrane of the white blood cell is usually highly convoluted and probably cannot carry large stresses in this state.

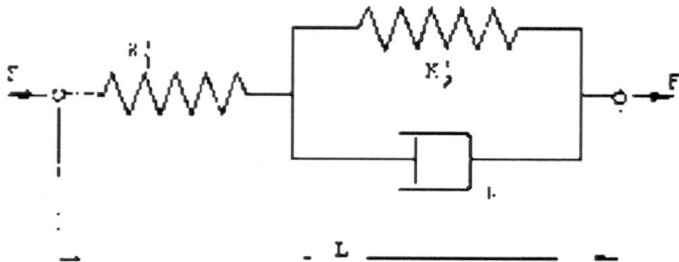

FIGURE 2. Standard solid model composed of a Kelvin body (K_2', μ) in series with a linear spring (K_1'). This model is equivalent to that shown in Fig. 1.

When applied to the cell as a whole in the glass capillary experiments the constants of the model in Fig. 1 will represent the combined behavior of the cytoplasm of the cell, the nucleus, the granules, and the membranes of the exterior surface, the nucleus and granules. Each of these components may in turn be representable by some similar viscoelastic model. At present insufficient information is available to model each constituent and to then derive from their combination the entire cell properties.

When the model in Fig. 1 is used to model experiments with small diameter pipettes (4) the constants are interpreted to represent primarily the cytoplasm properties. The same three element model as shown in Fig. 1 may be used, but in this case the constants K_1, K_2, and the viscosity μ represent the cytoplasm itself rather than gross cell properties.

The first approximation useful for white blood cell analysis is a uniform viscoelastic sphere having the rheological characteristics indicated by Fig. 1. This is the model that is used in analyzing the micropipette experiments in which the deformations are small and primarily involve the cytoplasm in the vicinity of the micropipette tip. The membrane may be discounted because it carries little stress. The presence of granules in the cytoplasm may also be discounted to first approximation because they represent a fairly dilute concentration of particles.

A second approximation of a white blood cell should consist of the viscoelastic sphere enclosed in an elastic membrane which would have a bimodular character. As long as the membrane is not completely smoothed out by the deformation, the stresses in it can probably be neglected. Once the membrane is stretched out it has a higher stiffness and can be treated to first approximation as a surface of constant area. The surface area of both the exterior surface of a leukocyte and the surface of the nucleus are both known to be approximately constant (5). In the theory the membrane may be replaced by an average surface which may stretch under small stress until the membrane is completely unfolded. After this point the membrane is very stiff and able to carry any isotropic stress up to the point of membrane fracture.

The next level of complexity that seems reasonable is to model the nucleus of the white blood cell in the same way as the cell itself above. That is the nucleus may be represented as a uniform viscoelastic sphere enclosed by a bimodular membrane. Typically the nuclear membrane is also convoluted and may be assumed to offer little resistance until it is smoothed out. The properties of the nucleus material itself should probably be different from that of the cytoplasm of the rest of the cell. It can be inferred directly from smears of white blood cells on glass slides and from observations in glass capillaries (2) that the nucleus of the white blood cell is stiffer than the cytoplasm surrounding the nucleus.

More detailed models may be envisioned in which the granules of the white cell are represented as viscoelastic particles enclosed in their own membrane and the actual distorted shape of the typical leukocyte nucleus is included in the description. Such detailed modelling does not seem warranted or possible at present.

The modelling discussed so far assumes that the white blood cells are passive. To model the active state it will be necessary to recognize at least two kinds of regions within the cell separated by a moving boundary. It may be sufficient to consider the properties of each region to be passive and uniform. On the moving boundary the properties of the material are assumed to change. The moving boundary problem involved is similar to that of the extension of a frozen region in a body of liquid. This type of modelling is discussed in (6).

2. ANALYSIS OF THE VISCOELASTIC MODEL

When a model such as shown in Fig. 1 is used to represent the entire white blood cell, say, in a situation such as the deformation during a blood smear in which the cell is flat-

tened, the force F in Fig. 1 represents the total squeezing
force (dynes) and the length L (cm) may be taken to be the
overall dimension of the cell measured in the direction of
the squeezing force. In this case the spring constants K_1,
K_2 have units of dyn/cm. The viscous coefficient μ in this
case will have units of dyn-sec/cm. Starting with the relation
of force to length or velocity for each element the equation
relating the overall force F to the overall change in length
ΔL may be derived as shown in (7), for example. The end result
may be written in the form

$$\dot{F} + F \frac{\mu}{K_2} = \Delta L K_1 + \dot{L}\mu (1 + \frac{K_1}{K_2}) \tag{1}$$

where $\dot{F}$, $\dot{L}$, represent the time rate of change of the force and
the velocity of extension respectively. The ΔL represents the
change in the length L from its equilibrium position. The
response characteristics of a viscoelastic material may be
conveniently summarized in terms of a creep compliance function
J(t) and a relaxation modulus Y(t) (7). The creep compliance
is the change of length with time that results when a unit
force is suddenly applied at time t = 0. For the sudden
application of any other force F_0 at time t = 0 the response
is proportional to the creep compliance function since the
system is linear, i.e.

$$\Delta L = F_0 J(t) = F_0 \frac{1}{K_1} [1-(1- \frac{K_1}{K_1 + K_2}) e^{-\alpha t}] \tag{2}$$

The time constant α in Eq. (2) is given by

$$\alpha = \frac{K_2 K_1}{(K_1 + K_2)\mu} \tag{3}$$

The relaxation modulus is defined as the force developed
when a unit deflection ΔL is suddenly applied to the model
at t = 0. For any other step deflection ΔL_0 the force
developed will be proportional Y(t) because of the linearity
of the system, i.e.

$$F = \Delta L_0 Y(t) = \Delta L_0 K_1 [1 - \frac{K_2}{K_1} e^{-\beta t}] \qquad (4)$$

where the time constant β is given by

$$\beta = K_2/\mu \qquad (5)$$

It may be seen that the time constant β is a measure of the speed with which a force developed by a step in the deflection ΔL relaxes to its final value. The time constant α, Eq. (3) is a measure of the time that the final deflection due to a given increment of loading takes to develop.

As an alternative to the creep compliance and relaxation functions the system may be described in terms of a complex compliance under oscillatory force or oscillatory displacement (7). This description is not developed here because there are no tests at present in which oscillatory stresses have been used to test white blood cell properties.

For an arbitrary specified time history of force $F(t)$ the response $\Delta L(t)$ may be computed by superposition of a large number of small force increments using the creep compliance function Eq. (2). The result is a so-called hereditary integral

$$\Delta L(t) = F_0 J(t) + \int_0^t J(t-t') \frac{dF}{dt'} dt' \qquad (6)$$

In a similar manner the response to an arbitrary specified strain history $\Delta L(t)$ is given by a hereditary integral using the relaxation modulus Eq. (4)

$$F(t) = \Delta L_0 Y(t) + \int_0^t \Delta Y(t-t') \frac{dL}{dt'} dt' \qquad (7)$$

The expressions given by the above equations (2,4,6,7) may be used to fit various experiments on white blood cells to derive the appropriate constants K_1, K_2, μ. This was carried out by Bagge (8) on the basis of tests of leukocytes forced through tapered glass capillaries.

When the model shown in Fig. 1 is applied as a three
dimensional continuum model of the cytoplasm of the cell itself rather than the whole cell, it is necessary to consider
that the model applies to components of the stress and strain
tensors rather than to any finite dimension or particular
force involved. Further it is necessary to recognize that
the cytoplasm of the typical cell is essentially incompressible
under normal circumstances. This means that the model of
Fig. 1 does not apply in purely hydrostatic, i.e. isotropic,
stress conditions, but that the model applies to the shear
or deviatoric part of the stress and strain.

These ideas are expressed in the usual stress-strain
vocabulary (9) using σ_{ij} for the stress tensor and e_{ij} for
the strain tensor where i and j may each have the values 1,
2 or 3 referring to Cartesian coordinates (x_1, x_2, x_3). The
isotropic part of the stress is what would normally be called
the pressure p in a fluid. Thus

$$p = -\frac{1}{3}\sigma_{kk} \tag{8}$$

The minus sign in Eq. (8) arises because stresses in a solid
are taken to be positive when tension but the pressure is
reckoned positive as compression. The deviatoric parts of
σ'_{ij} is defined as the original stress tensor σ_{ij} minus the
isotropic part, i.e.

$$\sigma'_{ij} = \sigma_{ij} - \frac{1}{3}\sigma_{kk}\delta_{ij} \tag{9}$$

where δ_{ij} is the Kronecker delta, equal to one for i = j and
zero otherwise.

The deviatoric part of the strain tensor e'_{ij} is defined
in a similar manner by

$$e'_{ij} = e_{ij} - \frac{1}{3}e_{kk}\delta_{ij} \tag{10}$$

In this case the isotropic part e_{kk} is zero because of the equation of conservation of mass for an incompressible material. For the viscoelastic model shown in Fig. 1 the corresponding three dimensional constitutive equation is

$$\sigma'_{ij} + \frac{\mu}{k_2} \dot{\sigma}'_{ij} = e'_{ij} k_1 + \dot{e}'_{ij} \mu (1 + \frac{k_1}{k_2}) \qquad (11)$$

where k_1 and k_2 are two elastic coefficients (dyn/cm^2) and μ is a coefficient of viscosity (dyn sec/cm^2). The $\dot{\sigma}'_{ij}$ and $\dot{e}'_{ij}$ indicate the time derivatives. Eq. (11) is of the same form as Eq. (1), but Eq. (11) applies to each component of the stress and strain tensors.

In order to solve problems using the viscoelastic model of Eq. (11) it is necessary to satisfy the equations of continuity and of equilibrium in addition to the constitutive equation (11). The solution to such problems can be cast in terms of an equivalent problem of a purely elastic material by the use of the so-called correspondence principle (7,9). The problem of the viscoelastic material response is converted into an analogous elastic problem by the use of the Laplace transform. The solution of the elastic problem is then carried out and an inverse Laplace transform is used to derive the final solution of the original viscoelastic problem. This procedure has been completely carried out for the case of a step pressure suddenly applied in the micropipette experiment in (4). The result is a stress field proportional to the stress that would be obtained if the cell were elastic multiplied by the creep function, $J(t)$, Eq. (2). This is the only case that has been carried out in detail in the literature, but in principle any case of small strains may be accomplished in this way.

3. DISCUSSION

The above discussion suggests the application of the linear theory of viscoelasticity assuming small strains can be profitably applied as a first approximation in the analysis of deformations of white blood cells. Numerical values of the material constants derived from micropipette experiments are given in a companion paper (10). To analyze large deformations such as occur in the tapered capillary experiment it would be necessary to extend the theory to the finite viscoelasticity equations involving large deformation. The next step in refinement of the theory will be to take into account the stress in the cell membrane. As the deformations become large and the membrane is stretched taut, these stresses will become more important. The tensile stress required to unfold corrugations of the membrane of the order of 0.4 μm in height and in width may be estimated by use of the elastica theory (11). The membrane is assumed to have a bending stiffness of 10^{-12} dyn/cm and to be locally of constant area (inextensible). Then the stress required to stretch the membrane taut is of the order of 0.02 dyn/cm. This may be contrasted to a fracture stress estimated to be approximately 5.0 dyn/cm. Between these two limits, the membrane will carry any isotropic stress applied with essentially constant area.

At present no large deformation results using three dimensional theory are available. The viscoelastic theory may also be used for the active deformation of white blood cells by postulating two different regions with different properties representing the normal cytoplasm and gelated pseudopods. This problem will also require large displacement theory if realistic pseudopods are to be generated.

ACKNOWLEDGEMENTS

This work was supported by U.S.P.H.S. Grant HL-16851 from the National Heart, Lung and Blood Institute.

REFERENCES

1. Branemark, P-I. 1971. Intravascular Anatomy of Blood
    Cells in Man. S. Karger, Basel, pp. 43-55.
2. Bagge, U., Skalak, R., Attefors, R. 1977. Granulocyte
    rheology. Advances in Microcirculation. $\underline{7}$:29-48.
3. Lichtman, M.A. 1973. Rheology of leukocytes, leukocyte
    suspensions and blood in leukemia. J. Clin. Invest.
    $\underline{52}$:350-358.
4. Schmid-Schonbein, G.W., Sung, K.L.P., Tozeren, H., Skalak,
    R., Chien, S. 1981. Passive mechanical properties of
    human leukocytes. Biophys. J., in press.
5. Schmid-Schonbein, G.W., Chien, S., Shih, Y.Y. 1980.
    Morphometry of human leukocytes. Blood. $\underline{56}$:866-875.
6. Schmid-Schonbein, G.W., Sung, K.L.P., Skalak, R., Chien,
    S. 1981. Human leukocytes in the active state. This
    Workshop.
7. Flugge, W. 1967. Viscoelasticity. Blaisdell Publishing
    Co., London.
8. Bagge, U. 1975. Experimental studies on the rheological
    properties of white blood cells in man and rabbit and in
    an in vitro micro-flow system. Doctoral dissertation,
    Department of Anatomy, University of Gothenburg, Sweden.
9. Fung, Y.C. 1965. Foundations of Solid Mechanics.
    Prentice-Hall, Englewood Cliffs, N.J.
10. Chien, S., Sung, K.L.P., Skalak, R., Schmid-Schonbein, G.W.
    1981. Viscoelastic properties of leukocytes in passive
    deformation. This Workshop.
11. Love, A.E.H. 1944. A Treatise on the Mathematical Theory
    of Elasticity. Dover Publications, New York, p. 401.

VISCOELASTIC PROPERTIES OF LEUKOCYTES IN PASSIVE DEFORMATION

S. CHIEN , K.L.P. SUNG , R. SKALAK , G.W. SCHMID-SCHÖNBEIN

1. INTRODUCTION

Knowledge on the rheological properties of white blood cells (WBCs) is essential for the understanding of their functional behavior in health and disease, including their deformation during release from the bone marrow, motion and deformation in blood vessels, rolling on the vascular endothelium, migration through the capillary wall into the interstitium, and deformation during phagocytosis. The viscoelastic properties of WBCs during large deformation have been investigated with the use of micropipettes (1, 2) and narrow glass capillaries (3). In such large deformations involving the whole cell, rheological measurements reflect the geometric features of the cell and the behavior of the nucleus, as well as the properties of the cytoplasm. This paper summarizes some results of our recent studies on the passive mechanical behavior of WBCs during small deformation in response to micropipette aspiration (4, 5, 6). The viscoelastic coefficients of the WBC derived from such small deformation data, with the aid of a theoretical model (7), reflect primarily the properties of the cytoplasm. In these experiments the use of EDTA, which causes chelation of Ca^{++}, serves to eliminate the active, spontaneous deformation of the WBC; such active mechanical properties of the WBC are discussed in an accompanying paper (8).

2. MATERIALS AND METHODS

Fresh blood samples were obtained from healthy human volunteers with EDTA as anticoagulant. The red blood cells were allowed to sediment at room temperature for 25-40 minutes, and the WBC-rich plasma was diluted with a pre-filtered, buffered saline-albumin solution to a concentration of about 50 WBCs/mm^3. The solution contained 0.9 g/dl NaCl, 0.25 g/dl bovine serum albumin, and 12 mM Tris, with pH adjusted to 7.4 by the dropwise addition of 1 N HCl. The studies were performed at 21-23°C, except in experiments in which the temperature was altered. Variations in osmolality of the medium was achieved by changing the concentration of NaCl, and alterations in pH were attained by changing the amount of Tris or HCl.

About 0.5-1 ml of the cell suspension was loaded in a small round chamber located on the stage of an inverted microscope. Individual WBCs were viewed with an 100x objective (NA 1.25, oil immersion) and a 20x eyepiece. The viewing field was displayed on a TV monitor through a video camera connected to the eyepiece, and the video image was recorded on a video recorder.

Micropipettes with internal radii of 1.1-1.7 μm were filled with the buffered saline-albumin solution and mounted on a hydraulic micromanipulator. The wide end of the micropipette was connected to a pressure regulation system. The pressure level was monitored with the use of a Statham transducer connected to a Gould recorder.

To analyze the time course of deformation of the neutrophils, sequential photographs were taken from the video image during single frame replay on the TV monitor. The displacement of the cell surface into the pipette was determined by subtracting the distance that the cell reaches into the pipette without deformation. The displacement data were entered into a PDP 11/10 minicomputer and analyzed by using our theoretical model (7), in which the neutrophil is treated as a standard solid consisting of an elastic element K_1 in parallel with a Maxwell element (an elastic element K_2 in series with a viscous element μ).

3. RESULTS

3.1. Time History of Neutrophil Deformation in Response to Aspiration Pressure.

Fig. 1 shows the time course of deformation of a neutrophil in saline-albumin solution (pH 7.4, 300 mOsm, 21-23°C) in response to an aspiration pressure (1 cm H_2O) applied via a micropipette. The WBC was rapidly displaced towards the pipette tip and sealed it within 1 or 2 television frames (16 to 32 msec). The first frame in which the WBC is seen to make contact with the pipette tip is denoted zero time (0 msec in Fig. 1). At this earliest detectable moment of contact, the WBC already underwent some deformation; the deformational entry of the WBC into the pipette

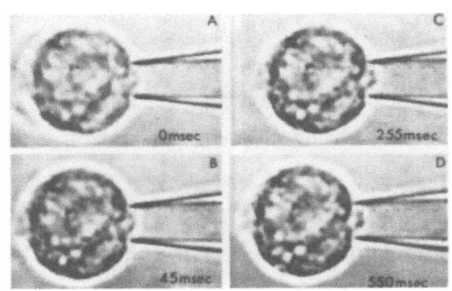

FIGURE 1. Photographs showing the time course of deformation of a human neutrophil in isotonic saline-albumin (300 mOsm, pH 7.4, 22°C). ΔP = 1000 dyn/cm^2.

showed an initial, rapid phase which was essentially synchronous with the applied pressure. This elastic response was followed by a creep displacement that was nonlinear with time. Fig. 2 shows the time histories of the aspiration pressure [$\Delta P(t)$] and cell displacement [$d(t)$] for a single neutrophil (pH 7.4, 511 mOsm, 22°C) subjected to three levels of ΔP. The continuous lines for $d(t)$ in Fig. 2 represent the best fit of the standard solid model (7) to the experimental data, and the coefficients K_1, K_2 and μ are listed in the figure. The general agreement of these coefficients among the three experiments supports the assumption of a linear relation, at any instant, between $d(t)$ and $\Delta P(t)$. Similar results were obtained for other neutrophils and at other osmolalities. In general, the linear assumption is satisfied when $d(t)$ is less than approximately 0.9 µm, but for larger deformations the model overestimates the experimental results.

14

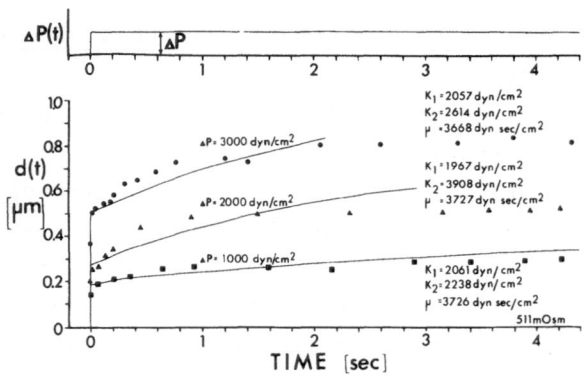

FIGURE 2. Time history of displacement [d(t)] for a neutrophil in hypertonic saline-albumin (511 mOsm, pH 7.4, 22°C) in
response to 3 different levels of aspiration pressure [ΔP].
The lines represent the best fit of the data with the standard
solid model using the coefficient K_1, K_2 and μ listed.

Another way to test the assumption of linearity as well as the
validity of the model is to apply, after the first pressure step
at t = 0, a second step at t > 0 with an additional ΔP. Fig. 3
shows the results of one such experiment (pH 7.4, 500 mOsm, 23°C).
The coefficients K_1, K_2 and μ were computed only for the first
step (for times t < 3 sec in Fig. 3). The theoretical line drawn
for the second step represents a prediction based on the coefficients derived from the first step. This prediction agrees well
with the experimental data obtained from the second step.

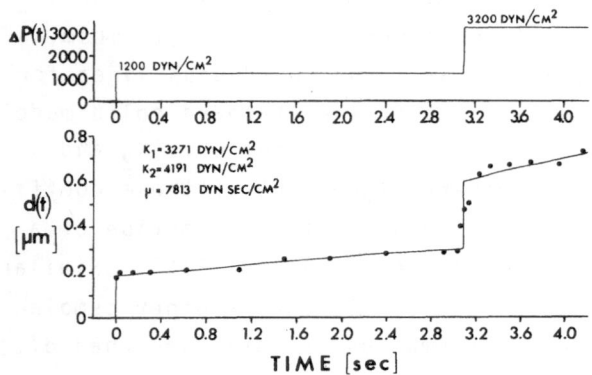

FIGURE 3. Two-step de-
formation of a neutro-
phil in hypertonic
saline-albumin (500
mOsm, pH 7.4, 23°C).
K_1, K_2 and μ
obtained from the first
step were used to
derive the line for the
second step.

The viscoelastic coefficients obtained on 75 neutrophils suspended in isotonic saline-albumin (pH 7.4, 310 mOsm, 21-23°C) are listed in Table I.

Table I. Viscoelastic Coefficients of Neutrophils*

Coefficients	Mean ± S.D.
K_1	275 ± 119 dyn/cm^2
K_2	737 ± 346 dyn/cm^2
μ	130 ± 54 dyn-sec/cm^2

*The neutrophils were suspended in isotonic saline-albumin solution (pH 7.4, 310 mOsm, 21-23°C). Number of neutrophils studied = 75. Values given are mean ± S.D.

3.2. Effects of Alterations in Physicochemical Factors on Viscoelastic Properties of Neutrophils.

3.2.1. Effects of temperature.

Over a temperature range of 9° to 40°C, the elastic constants (K_1 and K_2) of the neutrophil did not vary significantly with temperature. The μ value, however, varied inversely with temperature. The speed of Brownian motion of granules in the neutrophils varied directly with temperature.

3.2.2. Effects of pH variations.

The range of pH studied was 5.4 to 8.4. The K_2 values remained essentially constant in different pH media, but K_1 and μ increased with increasing pH. In the higher pH media (pH 7.8 and 8.4), the cell diameter increased, and the granules also became swollen.

3.2.3. Effects of variations in Osmolality.

The values of K_1, K_2 and μ increased nearly exponentially with increasing osmolality of the suspension medium in the range of 200 mOsm to 660 mOsm (data on μ are shown in Fig. 4). When the osmolality was reduced from 200 mOsm to 150 mOsm, K_2 increased slightly, but K_1 and μ did not show any significant change. The speed of Brownian motion of granules in the neutrophils varied inversely with osmolality. When a WBC has become

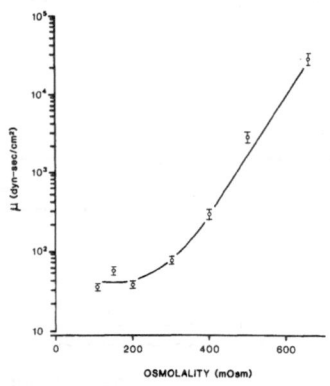

FIGURE 4. Effects of variations in osmolality on the viscosity (μ) of neutrophils. Vertical bars are standard errors of the mean.

swollen in an hypotonic medium, the two-step aspiration experiment shows that the deformation in the second step is generally overestimated by using the viscoelastic coefficients derived from the first step (Fig. 5). Under this condition the loss in excess membrane area (9) may favor the generation of significant membrane tension during micropipette aspiration and cause a nonlinearity in the relationship between $\Delta P(t)$ and $d(t)$.

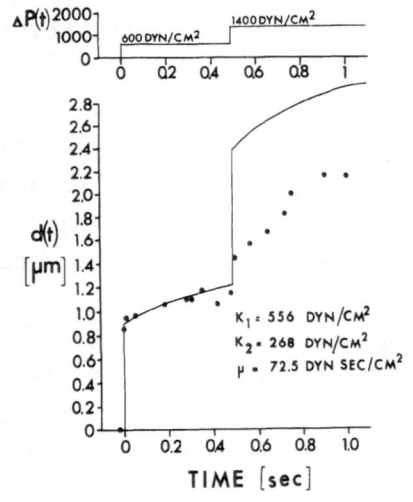

FIGURE 5. Two-step deformation of a neutrophil in hypotonic saline-albumin solution (200 mOsm, pH 7.4, 23°C). K_1, K_2 and μ were obtained by fitting the data in the first step with the use of the standard solid model. These coefficients were used to derive the line for the second step, resulting in an overestimation of the results.

In suspending media with an osmolality of 100 mOsm or less, WBC deformation in response to aspiration became limited as the cell was swollen to approach a smooth sphere (Fig. 6). This limited degree of deformation cannot be increased by raising the aspiration pressure, even up to 20,000 dyn/cm^2. At osmolalities < 100 mOsm, the data were variable because some of the WBCs underwent lysis after hypotonic swelling while others were fully or only partially swollen. Neutrophils that were tested in a 50 mOsm medium did not show any measurable deformation for all aspiration pressures that were applied without rupturing the membrane.

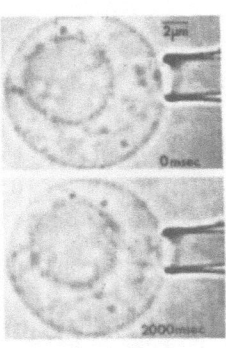

FIGURE 6. Two photographs showing a WBC swollen in hypotonic saline-albumin (108 mOsm, pH 7.4) to nearly spherical shape. Cell granules and nucleus are visible. The deformation was very small in response to a high ΔP value of 6000 dyn/cm^2; there was no detectable difference in the degree of deformation between 0 and 2 sec.

4. DISCUSSION

Our experiments on human neutrophils subjected to small deformations indicate that their cytoplasm behaves like a viscoelastic material whose main features can be modeled with a three-element standard solid material. The agreement between the model and data is good for small strains. For large deformations [d(t) > 0.9 μm] when some of the assumptions made in the modeling (7) are not applicable, the computed surface displacements overestimate the measured values. The standard solid model gives mean properties of the cell by averaging the stress over all cytoplasmic structures and the membrane. In an isotonic medium at physiological pH, when there exists a large (≃ 83 percent) excess membrane area (9), the contribution of the membrane to the viscoelastic behavior of the neutrophil during small deformation is probably negligible (7).

Previous workers (1, 2) have applied micropipette suction to study human leukocytes, but the design of their experiments is different from ours. They used pipettes with larger inner diameter (≃ 5 μm) to aspirate the entire cell inside the pipette and employed the pressure needed for this process as a measure of the elasticity of the cell. The overall cell geometry is an important factor in these studies. Furthermore, there may be an adhesive force between the tightly fitting cell and the inner wall of the pipette, when there is a large contact area between cell and glass.

With the use of a similar 3-element model in an one-dimensional strain analysis, Bagge et al. (3) deduced from their experimental study on grannulocyte deformation in a glass capillary with stenosis that $K_1 \simeq 3$ dyn/cm, $K_2 \simeq 30$ dyn/cm and $\mu \simeq 60$ dyn-sec/cm. These results cannot be compared directly with those obtained in the present study, but they probably represent higher viscoelastic moduli (4). The time constant of the WBC deformation process, which can be expressed as $\mu(K_1+K_2)/K_1K_2$, is on the order of 0.6 sec for the small deformation of WBC in the present study. In contrast, the time constant in large deformation of the entire WBC (3) is on the order of 20 sec. This discrepancy illustrates the difference in WBC properties when tested with a small deformation (the present study) and when examined with a large deformation of the whole cell (3). Deformation of the entire WBC may involve the nucleus and other structures with higher moduli, as well as the unfolding of the cell membrane; furthermore, there may be nonlinearity of the moduli in various components of the WBC.

Changes in rheological properties of neutrophils following alterations in physicochemical conditions can be demonstrated by the micropipette method. Over a temperature range from 9 to 40°C, the K_1 and K_2 values remain essentially constant, whereas the value of μ varies inversely with temperature, similar to the temperature dependence seen in other liquids and erythrocytes (10, 11). In experiments using suspending media with different pH, the cells show increases in K_1 and μ in alkaline solutions (pH 8.4). These rheological changes are associated with swelling of the cell and its granules and nucleus. The loss of cell membrane folding with neutrophil swelling would reduce the excessive membrane surface area available for deformation (9) and contribute to the observed changes in rheological properties.

In experiments using suspending media with different osmolalities, all three coefficients of neutrophils increase markedly in response to hypertonic shrinkage, probably reflecting the increase in solid concentration due to cellular dehydration. When the osmolality is reduced from 300 to 200 mOsm, there is a slight decrease in μ of neutrophils, as the cytoplasm is diluted with water. In 100 mOsm medium the cell has an almost spherical shape with unfolded membrane. The overall rheological properties of the neutrophil in response to variations in osmolality reflect a balance between the influences of the intracellular solid concentration and the geometric relation between cell surface area and volume. At low osmolalities near 200 mOsm, the relative constancy of the moduli values probably results from a balance of the decrease in solid concentration and the increase in sphericity, as the osmolality is lowered. At osmolalities of 100 mOsm or lower, when all the surface foldings in most cells disappear and the neutrophil becomes a smooth sphere, the cell becomes essentially non-deformable despite the increase in fluidity of the cell interior.

The value of μ for the normal WBCs is approximately 100 Poises, which is about 2000 times higher than the viscosity of the hemoglobin solution inside the red blood cell (RBC) (12). In addition, WBCs have about twice the volume of RBCs (9). Therefore, WBCs impose a much larger resistance in capillary blood vessels than RBCs (3). In hypotensive states this may lead to plugging of WBCs at the entrance to capillary vessels and thus cessation of flow (13). Due to the lower velocity of WBCs than RBCs in capillaries, a hydrodyamic collision follows which leads to regular attachment of WBCs on the venous endothelium (14). The relatively small deformation of the white cells on the venous endothelium with a major portion of the cell reaching into the flow field in venules causes a large elevation of the flow resistance in these vessels (15).

ACKNOWLEDGEMENTS

This work was supported by U.S.P.H.S. Grant HL-16851 from the National Heart, Lung and Blood Institute.

REFERENCES

1. Lichtman, M.A. 1973. Rheology of leukocytes, leukocyte suspensions and blood in leukemia. J. Clin. Invest. 52: 350-358.

2. Miller, M.E., Myers, K.A. 1975. Cellular deformability of the human peripheral blood polymorphonuclear leukocyte: Method of study, normal variation, effects of physical and chemical alterations. J. Reticuloendothel. Soc. 18: 337-345.

3. Bagge, U., Skalak, R., Attefors, R. 1977. Granulocyte rheology. Adv. Microcirc. 7:29-48.

4. Chien, S., Sung, K.L.P., Schmid-Schönbein, G.W., Tözeren, A., Tözeren, H., Usami, S., Skalak, R. 1980. Microrheology of erythrocytes and leukocytes. In Symposium on Hemorheology and Diseases (ed. J.F. Stoltz and P. Drouin), Doin Editeurs, Paris, pp.93-108.

5. Schmid-Schönbein, G.W., Sung, K.L.P., Tözeren, H., Skalak, R., Chien, S. 1981. Passive mechanical properties of human leukocytes. Biophys. J., in press.

6. Sung, K.L.P., Schmid-Schönbein, G.W., Skalak, R., Schuessler, G.B., Usami, S., Chien, S. 1981. Influence of physicochemical factors on rheology of human neutrophils. Blood, submitted for publication.

7. Skalak, R., Schmid-Schönbein, G.W., Chien, S. 1981. Analysis of white blood cell deformation. This Workshop.

8. Schmid-Schönbein, G.W., Sung, K.L.P., Skalak, R., Chien, S. 1981. Human leukocytes in the active state. This Workshop.

9. Schmid-Schönbein, G.W., Chien, S., Shih, Y.Y. 1980. Morphometry of human leukocytes. Blood, 56:866-875.

10. Handbook of Chemistry and Physics. 1962. Chemical Rubber Publishing Company, Cleveland, Ohio p. 2257.

11. Hochmuth, R.M., Buxbaum, K.L., Evans, E.A. 1980. Temperature dependence of the viscoelastic recovery of red cell membrane. Biophys. J. 29:177-182.

12. Cokelet, G.R., Meiselman, H.J. 1968. Rheological comparison of hemoglobin solutions and erythrocyte suspensions. Science 161:275-278.

13. Bagge, U., Amundson, B., Lauritzen, C. 1980. White blood cell deformability and plugging of skeletal muscle capillaries in hemorrhagic shock. Acta Physiol. Scand. 180:159-163.

14. Schmid-Schönbein, G.W., Usami, S., Skalak, R., Chien, S. 1980. The interaction of leukocytes and erythrocytes in capillary and postcapillary vessels. Microvasc. Res. 19:45-70.

15. Lipowsky, H.H., Usami, S., Chien, S. 1980. In vivo measurements of "apparent viscosity" and microvessel hematocrit in the mesentery of the cat. Microvasc. Res. 19: 297-319.

HUMAN LEUKOCYTES IN THE ACTIVE STATE

G.W. SCHMID-SCHÖNBEIN , R. SKALAK , K.L.P. SUNG , S. CHIEN

1. INTRODUCTION

Study of the rheological properties of leukocytes is a fascinating subject, because these cells can be observed in two different states. In the passive state, leukocytes are spherical and they deform only when an external stress is applied, such as plasma fluid stress or an adhesive stress to a substrate. Once the external stress is removed the cell returns to the spherical shape. Leukocytes circulating in the microcirculation or rolling on the venous endothelium are usually in the passive state (1,2). In the active state, leukocytes deform spontaneously without an external force acting on them other than a uniform hydrostatic pressure. Therefore, the required energy is supplied by the cell itself. The leukocytes develop membrane projections (pseudopods) which lead to irregular cell shapes (3). In the circulation leukocytes deform spontaneously when they migrate across the endothelial wall (4) or in a chemotactic gradient (5-7), and during phagocytosis (8).

The question arises what physical mechanism leads to the spontaneous deformation of the leukocytes and the displacement during migration on a substrate. In this report, some experimental results on the spontaneous deformation of cells in free suspension and their mechanical properties as

tested with a micropipette experiment will be presented.
The experiments have been performed on cells in free suspension without adhesion. The effects of a uniform and nonuniform adhesive stress to a substrate on the cell motion will
be discussed qualitatively. The latter case may explain the
directional displacement of leukocytes in a chemical gradient (6,7).

2.   EXPERIMENTAL METHODS

2.1 Cell Material
     Fresh venous blood samples (10 ml) from healthy human
subjects with heparin as a anticoagulant were allowed to
sediment for ~40 min. The supernatant plasma layer containing leukocytes, platelets, and a few erythrocytes were collected and suspended in 10 ml Ringer solution.

2.2 Light Microscopy (LM)
     About 2 ml of leukocyte suspension was placed on a
round chamber which was mounted on the heated stage ($34^{O}C$)
of an inverted microscope. Single cells were viewed with a
100x objective (NA = 1.32, oil immersion) and a 25x eyepiece.
The image was recorded with a video camera, stored for
single frame replay on a video tape recorder system and displayed on a monitor. The final magnification (~5000x) was
established with a microscale (American Optics; 2 mm, 10 μm
div.) and time was recorded with a video timer. In order to
prevent sedimentation a gentle stream of fluid was ejected
from a micropipette adjacent to the leukocyte under observation. The pipette was positioned with a micromanipulator.
This procedure prevented cell attachment to the glass surface while keeping the leukocyte in focus.

2.3 Transmission and Scanning Electron Microscopy (TEM,SEM)
     Leukocytes in the active state were fixed with glutar-
aldehyde and post-fixed in OsO_4 in the same way as described
earlier for leukocytes in the passive state (9). The cells
were dehydrated with ethanol and embedded in araldite resin
for observation of thin sections with the TEM (Zeiss EM 9S2).

For investigation with the SEM (Jeol Corp.), cells in ethanol were dried with a critical point drying apparatus and
coated with gold palladium (for details see Ref. 9).

2.4 Micropipette Aspiration Experiment

Micropipettes with internal radius between 1.1 and 2.0
μm were filled with Ringer's solution and connected to a
pressure regulator. With this regulator a step pressure
could be applied to the cell surface, and by means of the
LM technique (see above) the resulting deformation history
of the cell could be observed. This is the same experimental technique as applied to the cells in the passive state
(10).

3. RESULTS

The discussion will be limited to neutrophils, but
similar observations were made with other leukocytes, unless
indicated otherwise.

3.1 Time Course of Leukocyte Deformation in the Active
State

Figure 1 shows a time sequence of neutrophils during
pseudopod formation as observed with the LM. The cell is in
free suspension and each photograph has been reoriented so
that the cell is shown without whole body rotation during
the observation period of ~130 sec. Figure 2A shows the
corresponding time sequence as measured by the length across
cell and pseudopod (L_1,L_2). The cell has been in Ringer
solution for 2 hours and 15 minutes after the phlebotomy.
The time sequence shows that the pseudopods form and retract
in cycles and they cause a nonsymmetric deformation of the
cell. During a growth period (from ~30 sec to 70 sec for
L_2 in Figure 2A) the pseudopod is devoid of all granules but
during the retraction period the granules are observed to
return by Brownian motion back into the pseudopod. The cell
may have at any time more than one pseudopod (Figure 2B).
We could not detect a regular pattern with respect to the
location of the pseudopods on the cell surface. At an early

time after the phlebotomy (~1 hr) the majority of the leukocytes have small pseudopods. At later times their size increases and the cells do not return to their undeformed
spherical shape. Neutrophils frequently form a neck which
originates at the pseudopod (Figure 3A) and which travels
along the main cell body with a speed of about 5.6 µm/min
(Figure 3B).

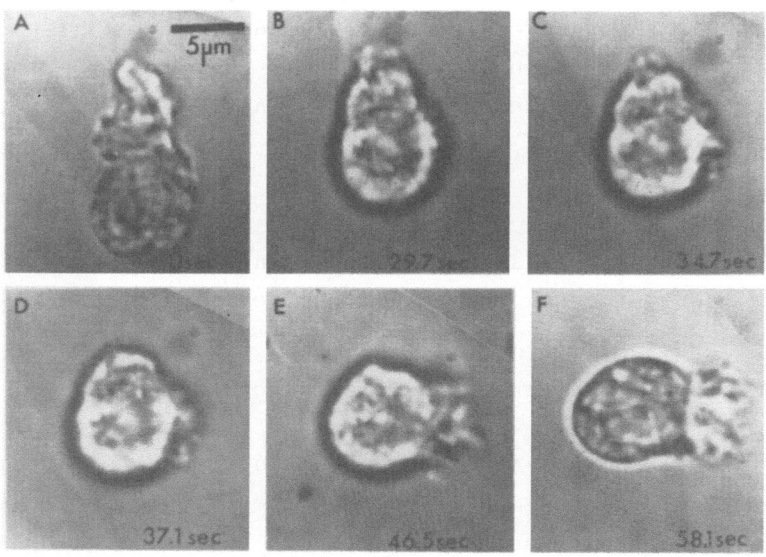

FIGURE 1. Sequence of photographs from the TV monitor showing the retraction (A-C) and formation (D-F) of pseudopods
on a human neutrophil in free suspension.

3.2 Electron Microscopic Investigation

Figure 4 shows several examples of neutrophils fixed in
the active state and viewed with the TEM. In the main cell
body one finds the usual cytoplasmic organelles whereas in
the pseudopod there is a striking exclusion of all organelles.
This agrees with the LM observation of a uniform clear cytoplasm in the pseudopod. The cell membrane around the main
cell body contains initially the same numerous fine folds as
seen on leukocytes in the passive state (Fig. 4A). As the
pseudopods grow in size these membrane folds are stretched
out (Fig. 4A). Under high magnification the material in the

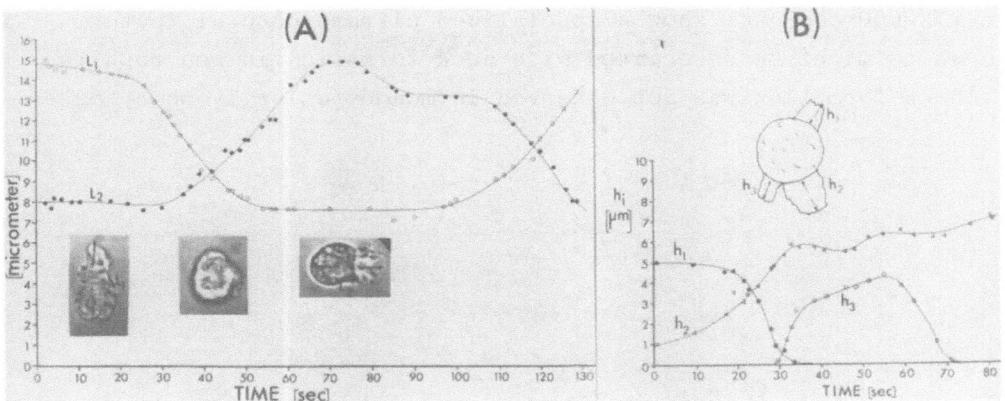

FIGURE 2. A) Time course of pseudopod formation (same cell as in Figure 1) as measured by the length L_1 and L_2 shown in the inserts. B) Pseudopod formation on a neutrophil in free suspension. The extension h_i of each pseudopod has been measured from the undeformed spherical shape.

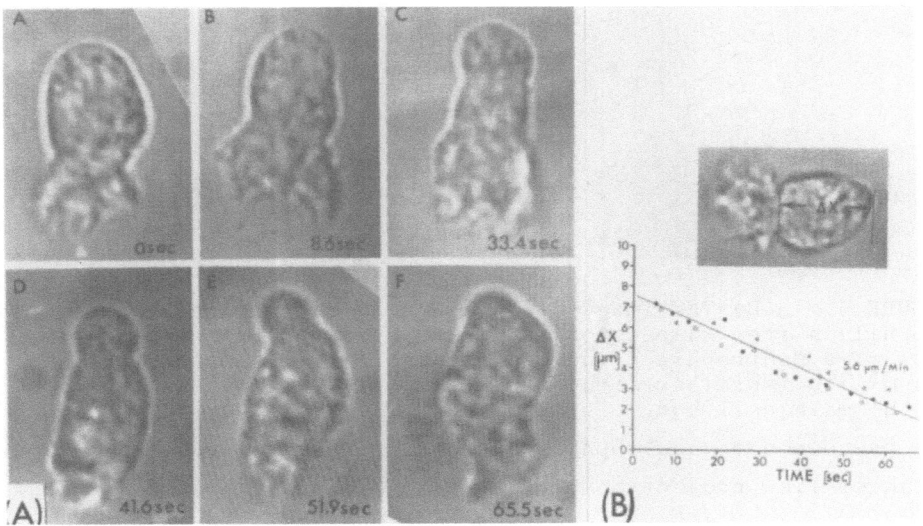

FIGURE 3. A) Sequence of photographs of a neutrophil with formation of a neck. B) The displacement ΔX of the neck as function of time. The different symbols refer to three subsequent cycles of pseudopod formation on the same cell. In all three cycles the pseudopod grew at the same location on the cell surface.

pseudopod shows a fine polymerized fibrillar structure (Fig. 4C). Figure 4D shows a cross section through a neutrophil with the characteristic neck as seen in LM (Fig. 3).

26

Observation of the neck region at magnifications up to x120000 does not show a specialized ultrastructural feature which might be associated with neck formation in neutrophils. Neck formation was not observed in monocytes or lymphocytes.

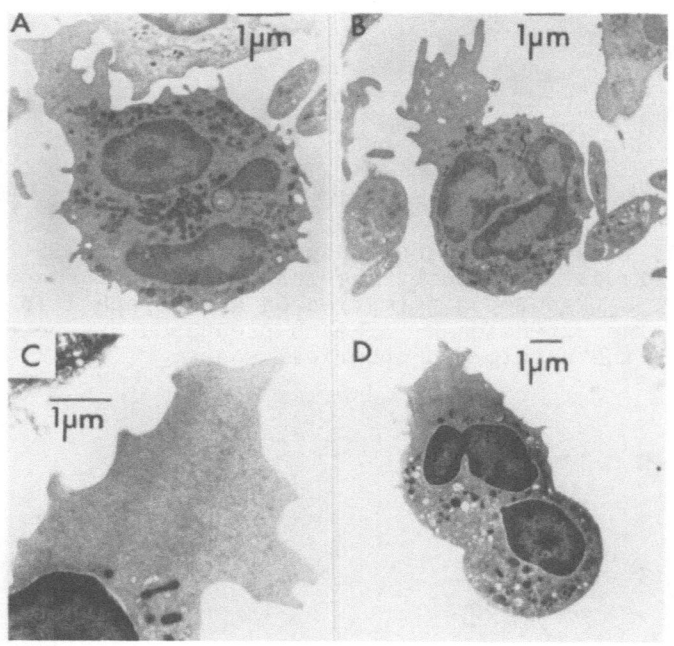

FIGURE 4. A,B) TEM image of a thin section throughout a neutrophil in free suspension with pseudopod. C) High power view of a neutrophil pseudopod showing a homogeneous cytoplasm with fibrillar structure. D) Neutrophil with a neck at the main cell body, as seen in LM (Fig. 3).

The pseudopod of neutrophils has usually several veil-like or sheet-like projections (Fig. 5). These sheet-like projections appear in thin sections as fingerlike projections (Fig. 4B). The membrane around each veil is unfolded and smooth. The pseudopods with polymerized cytoplasmic structure are always observed adjacent to the cell membrane, never in the interior of the cell.

3.3 Rheological Properties of Leukocytes in the Active State

The rheological properties of cell and pseudopod were compared by applying the micropipette aspiration pressure

either at the main cell body (Fig. 6A) or directly at a small
pseudopod (Fig. 6B). In both cases the aspiration pressure
ΔP was 800 dyn/cm^2 but the resulting deformation d(t) was
different. The deformation at the main cell body (Fig. 7A
open symbols) shows the typical nonlinear creep that one
sees in these cells, and the deformations at different points
on the cell are very similar. This indicates rather homogeneous mechanical properties of the cytoplasm in the main

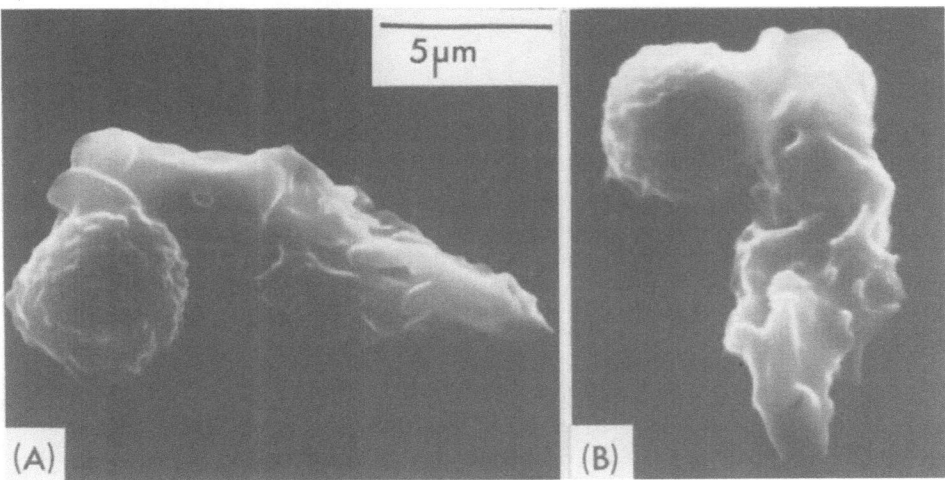

FIGURE 5. SEM view of the front (A) and side (B) of neutrophil in the active state. The cell was in free suspension
at the time of fixation. The pseudopod has veil-like projections each of which has a smooth membrane, and the main
cell body has the usual fine membrane folds. Note that leukocytes shrink significantly when dehydrated for SEM (9).

cell body, as it was seen in the passive state (10). On the
other hand, the deformation in the region of the pseudopod
is significantly smaller (Fig. 7A, filled symbols) and shows
only a small creep. This suggests that the polymerized cell
matrix in the pseudopod region has stiffer elastic mechanical
properties than the viscoelastic properties of the main cell
body with the cell organelle. When the cell is aspirated
at a pseudopod (Fig. 7B) one observes, after the initial
elastic response, the nonlinear creep deformation at the
time when the pseudopod retracts (about 6 sec in Fig. 7B).

28

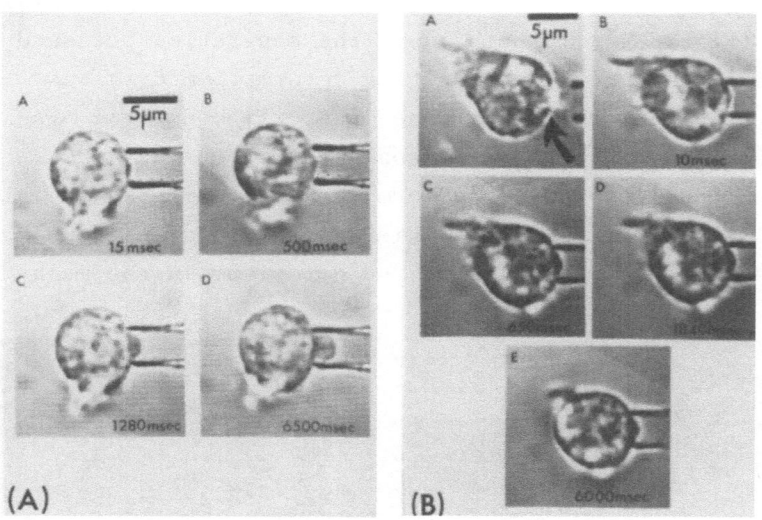

(A)

(B)

FIGURE 6. Sequence of photographs from the TV monitor showing a leukocyte deformation into the pipette in response to
a step aspiration pressure (800 dyn/cm^2). A) Aspiration at
the main cell body away from the pseudopod. B) Aspiration
of a small pseudopod (arrow).

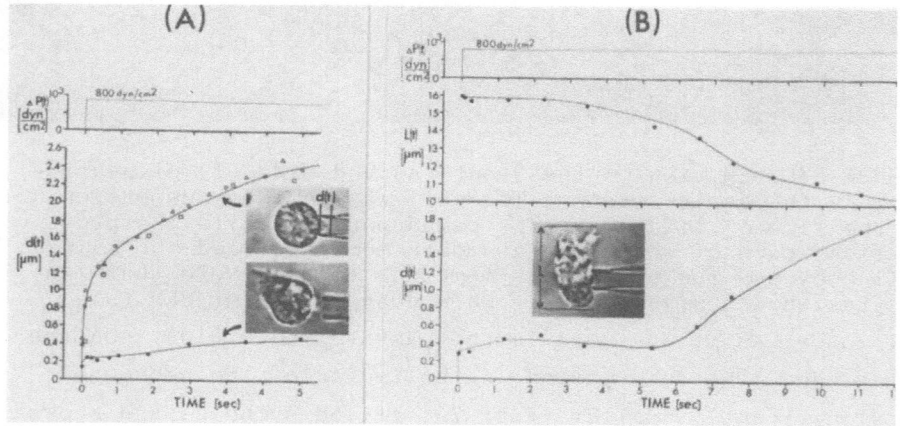

FIGURE 7. A) Micropipette aspiration pressure $\Delta P(t)$ and deformation $d(t)$ for a cell which was aspirated at the main
cell body (open symbols) and at a small pseudopod (closed
circles). B) The aspiration pressure $\Delta P(t)$, length of cell
and pseudopod $L(t)$, and deformation $d(t)$ into the pipette
for a neutrophil with retracting pseudopod. The lines were
drawn by hand.

4. DISCUSSION

The observations presented here suggest that leukocytes in the active state undergo a cyclic polymerization and depolymerization of their cytoplasm with the exclusion of all cell organelle from the polymerized cell matrix. The newly forming pseudopod consists of an arrangement of sheet-like projections, each of which has an unfolded membrane. This projection of the cell cytoplasm beyond the perimeter of the undeformed spherical cell seems to be the basic mechanism leading to displacement of the cell when it adheres to a substrate. On freely suspended leukocytes in uniform Ringer solution we cannot detect a preferential direction in which pseudopods are projected.

Morphometric analysis of neutrophils has shown that only 37% of the cell volume is occupied by the nucleus, granules, and mitochondria, whereas the majority of 63% is made up of the relative homogeneous cell matrix (9). Biochemical analysis of cell matrix extracts of horse leukocytes (11), guinea pig granulocytes (12), and rabbit macrophages (13) indicates that actin-like and myosin-like proteins and other high molecular components are present. These extracts appear to be able to gel (14) and change mechanical properties. Formation of the polymerized region in leukocytes is always initiated at the cell membrane suggesting that the polymerization is initiated by transport of a mediator, such as Ca^{++}, across the membrane. It is not clear presently what agent causes the depolymerization of the cell matrix at a retracting pseudopod.

To conlude, we discuss briefly the effects of an adhesive stress when the cell comes in contact with a substrate and forms a contact area. The adhesive stress may be uniform over the contact area or it may be nonuniform. This case may exist for example in the presence of a gradient of an adhesion causing substance. In the case of a uniform adhesive stress the cell will spread to increase its contact area with the substrate. Passive leukocytes will form a circular contact area (15). In face of the constant membrane

area of the cell (9) the maximum extent of spreading is
limited by the available membrane area. In the presence of
pseudopod formation the cell will form new contact area at
the advancing pseudopod and, in the presence of uniform adhesive stress, will break away with equal probability at any
point in the contact area. Thus the resulting displacement
of the cell will have a direction which is only dependent on
the direction in which the new pseudopods grow.

However, in the presence of a nonuniform adhesive stress
during formation of a new pseudopod the cell will break away
at the point of the weakest adhesive stress and the pseudopod will make new contact at a point of stronger adhesion to
the substrate. By repeating this process the cell will be
displaced in the overall direction of an increasing adhesive
stress. This is not necessarily dependent on the direction
in which the pseudopods grow, because the membrane which is
projected by the advancing pseudopod will apply tension at
all points of attachment to the substrate, but will break
only at the point of weakest attachment. This process will
continue until the adhesive stress is so strong that the
stress generated by an advancing pseudopod is insufficient
to break the bonds between cell and substrate in the entire
contact area. In this case the cell will stop to migrate.
This may be the mechanism by which leukocytes "sense" a
chemical gradient as seen in experiments on chemotaxis (5,6,
7). The observations presented here form a basis to a continuum mechanical theory of leukocytes in the active state
which will be presented later.

REFERENCES
1. Bagge U, Brånemark P-I. 1977. White blood cell rheology.
   An intravital study in man. Adv. Microcirc. 7: 1-17.
2. Schmid-Schönbein GW, Usami S, Skalak R, Chien S. 1980.
   The interaction of leukocytes and erythrocytes in capillary and postcapillary vessels. Microvasc. Res. 19: 45-
   70.
3. Lichtman MA, Santillo PA, Kearney EA, Roberts GW, Weed
   RI. 1976. The shape and surface morphology of human leukocytes in vitro: Effect of temperature, metabolic inhibitors and agents that influence membrane structure.
   Blood Cells, 2: 507-531.

4. Marchesi VT, Florey HW. 1960. Electron micrographic observations on the emigration of leukocytes. Quart. J. Exp. Physiol. 45: 343-347.
5. Gallin JI, Quie PG (editors). 1978. Leukocyte Chemotaxis: Methods, Physiology, and Clinical Implications. Raven Press, New York.
6. Wilkinson PC. 1974. Chemotaxis and Inflammation. Churchill Livingstone, Edinburgh and London.
7. Zigmoid SH. 1978. Chemotaxis by polymorphonuclear leukocytes. J. Cell Biol. 77: 269-287.
8. Elsbach P. 1974. Phagocytosis. In: The Inflammatory Process. BW Zweifach, L Grant, RT McCluskey (eds). Academic Press, Inc., New York. 2nd Edition 1: 363-410.
9. Schmid-Schönbein GW, Shih YY, Chien S. 1980. Morphometry of human leukocytes. Blood 56: 866-875.
10. Schmid-Schönbein GW, Sung KLP, Tözeren H, Skalak R, Chien S. 1981. Passive mechanical properties of human leukocytes. Biophys. J. 36: in press.
11. Shibata N, Takubo T, Senda N. 1979. Ca^{2+}-sensitive contractile protein from leucocytes. In: Cell Motility: Molecules and Organelle. S Hatano, H Ishikawa, H Sato (eds). University Park Press, Baltimore, pp. 13-31.
12. Stossel TP, Pollard TD. 1973. Myosin in polymorphonuclear leukocytes. J. Biol. Chem. 248: 8288-8294.
13. Hartwig JH, Stossel TP. 1975. Isolation and properties of actin, myosin, and a new actin binding protein in rabbit alveolar macrophages. J. Biol. Chem. 250: 5696-5705.
14. Brotschi EA, Hartwig JH, Stossel TP. 1978. The gelation of actin by actin-binding protein. J. Biol. Chem. 253 8988-8993.
15. Michaelis TW, Larrimer NR, Metz EN, Balcerzak SP. 1971. Surface morphology of human leukocytes. Blood 37: 23-30.

ACKNOWLEDGEMENT

This work was supported in part by NHLBI Research Grant HL 16851 and by a grant from the Office of Graduate Studies and Research at the University of California, San Diego. The excellent typing by Karen Kosakowski is greatly appreciated.

MECHANICAL BEHAVIOR OF LEUKOCYTES IN THE PASSIVE AND ACTIVE
STATES (COMMENTARY)

Giles R. Cokelet

As indicated by their coauthorship, the first three papers
presented at this workshop are the result of the close collaboration between Drs. Richard Skalak, Shu Chien, and Geert Schmid-
Schönbein, and their coworkers. The benefits of such interactive
cooperation between individual experts in complementary fields are
demonstrated in the contents of these presentations.
     In the first paper, Dr. Skalak has summarized the theoretical
aspects of research on the mechanical properties and behavior of
leukocytes (WBC). Several models of the WBC are discussed. The
first mathematical model is a phenomenological model which can be
used in two ways: (a) to represent the temporal relationship between some characteristic dimension (such as WBC length) and an
external force causing whole WBC deformation, or (b) to represent
the mechanical response of a differential volume of material,
such as cytoplasm, to a tension. The elements of this mathematical model probably do not have physical counterparts in the rea
WBC when the model is used to describe whole-cell deformation.
Consequently, the physical constants of this model, as found for
example in equation (1), may be dependent not only on the material
properties of the cell constituents, but also on cell geometry,
method and scale of deformation, etc. Nevertheless, the model can
be used to correlate data from similar tests.
     When equation (1) is used to describe the behavior of an
elemental volume of material, one must construct (mathematically)
an additional model if one wishes to relate the constants in the
equation to the observed mechanical deformation of all or part of
a cell. The simplest way to do this is to imagine that the cell
can be modelled as an initially spherical body of homogeneous
material whose properties are given by equation (1), and to derive

the equations which describe the response of this body to external forces. By fitting the observed behavior to the predictions of the whole cell model, one can evaluate the constants in equation (1). These constants may not be directly associated with real constituents within the cell.

Obviously, in the case of a heterogeneous cell, a model cell composed of a single homogeneous material can not be expected to represent the behavior of the real cell. However, under special test conditions, the response of a real cell may be due almost entirely to the response of a single phase or constituent located in a small part of the cell; then the response of the real cell may be interpreted with the homogeneous material mathematical model to obtain the mechanical properties of one constituent of the cell. This latter utility is exemplified by the analysis of data obtained during small scale deformation of WBC by aspiration of WBC into very small micropipettes (results presented by Dr. Shu Chien in the second paper).

Under the conditions of that test, the response of the cell is interpreted as reflecting primarily the properties of the cyto-plasm on the basis the (a) the WBC membrane is folded and until it is unfolded does not carry any stress, (b) the cell nucleus is not deformed and is far enough away from the test site so that it does not influence the test results, and (c) the granules are present only at such a low concentration as to not influence the test.

As shown by Dr. Chien in his presentation, this simple model represents the micropipette data obtained in a variety of tests on WBC remarkably well: the model is less successful in predicting WBC behavior at long times in creep tests (perhaps because of in-volvement of the cell nucleus and/or membrane stress) and in two-step tests involving WBC in hypotonic saline (because of signif-icant membrane stress in the unfolded membrane of the swollen cell). The phenomenological nature (in a general sense) of this simple mathematical model is pointed out by Dr. Chien by his com-parison of creep compliance time constants calculated from the model for small deformation of WBC and for whole cell deformation: about 0.6 seconds for small deformation and about 20 seconds for whole cell deformation.

Dr. Marshall Lichtman indicated that at least some WBC (e.g. lymphocytes) may have villi in the membrane folds and that therefore the membrane folds might not be unfoldable. If true, then the mathematical model constant would reflect a contribution from the membrane as well as from the cytoplasm.

Dr. Skalak has also outlined how one might proceed to progressively develop models which are more realistic in the sense that identifiable constituents of the cell are each represented in the mathematical model by specific material constants. The complexity of the mathematical development may approach the complexity of the real cell!

Dr Chien's paper describes how micropipettes with internal diameters of 2.2 - 3.4 microns were used to obtain data on the small deformation behavior of neutrophils; these data were obtained with WBC obtained from human blood collected with EDTA as the anticoagulant; the WBC were initially suspended in a buffered NaCl solution containing 0.25% bovine serum albumin (and a small amount of human plasma). The use of EDTA to chelate c cium ions keeps the WBC in their "passive" state, which is apparently the usual state of WBC while they are in the circulation. Some of these data were used to test the applicability of the mathematical model discussed above and the remaining data were used to demonstrate how the mechanical properties of cytoplasm change with temperature, pH, and osmolality.

A number of questions were discussed at the end of Dr. Chien presentation. Dr. U. Bagge asked if EDTA affects WBC deformability. Dr. Chien indicated EDTA was used because it kept the WBC in the inactive (passive) state; Dr. Geert Schmid-Schönbein said that when heparin is used as the anticoagulant, the WBC appear to be stiffened. In response to another question, Dr. Chien said that the WBC nucleus membrane is normally also folded and not a smooth surface. And to a wondering of why WBC seem to tolerate low pH and osmolality conditions much better than high values of these parameters, Dr. La Celle suggested that at least some WBC constituents undergo conformational changes when placed in the indicated high pH and osmolality environments.

In the third presentation, Dr. Geert Schmid-Schönbein described his observations on leukocytes (mostly neutrophils) which
were in the "active" state; by "active" state it is meant that
the WBC spontaneously (without the influence of external forces)
develop "sheet-like" extensions (pseudopods) over a time period
of the order of 20 - 40 seconds which then retract after a period
of time. These active WBC were obtained by collecting human blood
with heparin as the anticoagulant, separating the WBC by gravity
sedimentation and suspending the WBC at low concentration in
Ringer's solution (apparently without albumin) - the WBC become
active after standing at $37^{\circ}C$ for about 1 hour.

To this commentator, who knows nothing about such spontaneous
cellular activity, the observations were very interesting and
raised many questions, some of which are presented here.

1. Dr. Schmid-Schnönbein postulates a cyclical polymerization
-depolymerization of cytoplasm constituents as the mechanism causing pseudopod extension and retraction. To one whose schooling
included study of manmade polymers, the process of polymerization
and depolymerization involves the breaking and making of primary
molecular bonds, with large energy transfers. It is not clear
to this commentator what evidence supports the hypothesis that
the formation of pseudopods involves primary bond changes. Mechanisms based on molecular conformational changes and phase trans-
itions would seem to be equally likely candidates. The presence
of a fibrillar structure in the pseudopods shown in Figure 4 seems
ambiguous, but the commentator pleads guilty to the charge of not
being experienced in reading electron micrographs.

2. The absence of granules in the pseudopod implies a pseudopod growth mechanism which "extrudes" granules as the pseudopod
grows. This seems to imply a process which originates at the tip
of the pseudopod and which propagates backwards towards the WBC
main body. Could not this process involve the drawing towards
each other of opposing WBC membranes by a contractile mechanism
within the cytoplasm during a conformational transition of the
cytoplasm constituents?

3. In a freely-suspended stationary body, subject to zero
net external force, the center of mass of the body must remain

stationary as the body changes shape. Since the center of mass of the WBC can not be tracked (and the cell appears to move), it is difficult to say whether the pseudopod pushes itself out of the cell or if the tip of the pseudopod remains stationary relative to the WBC center of mass. If the WBC is attached to a surface, then an external force can be exerted on the WBC and its center of mass can move during pseudopod formation.

4. The micorpipette studies of active WBC are very interesting. The response difference seen when micropipette aspiration is applied to a portion of the WBC near a pseudopod rather than to a portion of the WBC far from a pseudopod is very striking. A direct comparison between the results for inactive WBC (reported by Dr. Chien) and for active WBC regions far away from the pseudopod can not be made from these presentations; the figures of deformation distance-time curves in Dr. Chien's presentation are for WBC in abnormal environments, and alternatively, one does not have the mathematical model needed for predicting the deformation distance-time behavior on normal passive WBC from the viscoelastic constants in Table I of Dr. Chien's paper. It would be very informative to have this comparison in quantitative terms

Dr. Schmid-Schönbein concludes his presentation with a discussion of how pseudopod behavior and cell adhesion to surfaces might lead to cell migration. This part of his presentation generated considerable discussion. Among the comments was one made by Dr. Wilkinson to the effect that some chemotactic agents reduce WBC adhesion to surfaces and so a WBC migrating along a gradient in agent concentration would also be migrating along a gradient of decreasing adhesion, which is not an observation which is easily incorporated into the hypothesis presented by Dr Schmid-Schönbein. Dr. Wilkinson also observed that pseudopods separate from WBC and that these separated pseudopods also migrate in a gradient of chemotactic agent. Dr. Lackie indicated that the most closely attached part of the migrating cell was the moving part of the cell (as determined by an interference reflection method) which seemed contrary to the expectations of Dr. Schmid-Schönbein Another interesting observation reported by Dr. Wilkinson was that the "neck" which Dr. Schmid-Schönbein described as travelling

from the pseudopod across the main body of the WBC travels in
an apparently different manner on cells attched to surfaces: the
"neck" remains stationary and the WBC moves through the "neck".

Taken as a whole, these three papers summarized the results
obtained in investigation of the mechanical properties and behavior of WBC by the use of methods well established in erythrocyte studies but which have only recently been applied to the
WBC. The application of these findings to biologically important
WBC processes is new and as a result is somewhat controversial and
unsettled. The three authors are to be congratulated for their
innovative approach to studying the WBC, and it is hoped that
cooperation and interaction with those who have a large background
in, for example, the biochemistry of WBC, chemotaxis and amoeboid
motion will lead to a rapid advancement in our understanding of
how WBC move.

VISCOELASTIC PROPERTIES OF NORMAL AND PATHOLOGIC HUMAN GRANULOCYTES AND LYMPHOCYTES

P.L. LA CELLE, R.W. BUSH, B.D. SMITH

1. INTRODUCTION

Leukocytes differ significantly from normal erythrocytes in cytostructure, characteristics of plasma membrane, relative sphericity in vivo, and in phagocytic types, the energy dependent mechanisms which permit motility and phagocytosis. Their rheologic behavior in vivo differs importantly from that of erythrocytes (1-3), flow is significantly slower (2) and the interactions of leukocytes with endothelium and erythrocytes influence blood flow (2,3). Granulocytes and lymphocytes can traverse capillaries of 4-8 μm dia. at relatively low pressures (3) however individual cells may obstruct flow at forces exceeding those in capillaries, with resulting obstruction presumed to be due to the leukocytes' relative sphericity, surface properties in relation to endothelial cells, positioning in the flow and unknown factors. Pathologic cells from leukemic states are presumed to affect blood rheology adversely because of abnormalities of cell deformability associated with atypical cell development (4). The present study examines the viscoelasticity of normal and pathologic human granulocytes and lymphocytes by observations of deformation of cells in micropipettes and in flow channels; investigates the effects of temperature; and records the relative adherence of these cells to endothelium to provide comparison with the well known properties of the human erythrocyte. Results were compared with earlier results obtained for deformation of normal white cells in well defined low shear fields in a parallel plate flow channel (5).

2. PROCEDURE

Material and methods

Cells. Normal and leukemic human granulocytes and lymphocytes were obtained from fresh human blood samples made calcium-poor by chelation, and individual cell types were concentrated by elutriation, standard gradient and filtration methods. Cells for study were suspended in phosphate buffer containing 0.5 g/dl autologous plasma and EGTA 0.1 g/dl. Observations of cell deformation were made by use of an inverted microscope and video system, with provision of video tape recording for subsequent analysis.

Micropipette deformation. The membrane and adjacent underlying cytoplasm of granulocytes and lymphocytes were aspirated in 1 to 1.5 μm diameter glass micropipettes with 1000 dyn/cm^2 increments of pressure over the range 0-10000 dynes/cm^2 in 5 minutes and the length of aspirated membrane D divided by pipette radius R_p related to applied pressure times pipette radius. The linear portion was utilized for comparisons. The cellular deformability, estimated by recording pressures to aspirate entire cells into 2.5 to 4.6μ m micropipettes over a 30 second period was measured for granulocytes and lymphocytes. Recovery of deformed portions of cytoplasm and extensional recovery of cells were observed as a function of time for lymphocytes, by the techniques described earlier (6,7).

Flow channel experiments. Flow channels suitable for microscope stage were prepared such that channel depth was 0.0 125cm and pressure drop across the channel could be monitored by a pressure transducer (8). Cells introduced were allowed to settle for 30 min. the channel flushed and deformation of individual cells attached by single points were observed as a function of increments of flow rate. Cells were compared in terms of deformation (length, 1/initial length, l_o) vs τ_W, the fluid shear stress at the chamber surface (8).

Temperature experiments. Recovery of deformed
lymphocytes and granulocytes was observed at 37°C as well as
at room temperature (20°C) and 25°C.

Force for detachment of leukocytes from endothelial
cells. Monolayer cultures of human cord endothelial cells were
prepared on plastic chambers and lymphocytes and granulocytes
were introduced and allowed to settle for thirty minutes.
Shear stress for detachment was measured at 25°C for normal
lymphocytes and granulocytes with normal erythrocytes as
controls.

3. RESULTS

Micropipette deformation experiments. Data obtained in
deformation of leukocytes is presented in Table 1 in terms of
deforming pressure required to achieve a standard hemispherical
displacement of membrane and contiguous cytoplasm in the
pipette tip.

Table 1

Deformation of normal and pathologic leukocytes

Cell type	Comparative deforming pressure* $P \cdot R_p$ (dyn/cm) X 10^3	
	20°C	37°C
Neutrophilic granulocyte	15	12
Lymphocyte	20	18
CML granulocyte	14	–
AML myeloblast	23	–
CLL lymphocyte	21	–
Lymphoblast	23	–
Normal erythrocyte	3	2

*for standard deformation $D/R_p = 0.5$

Because lymphocytes and granulocyts possess appxoximately 60 to
80% excess membrane area over that required to enclose their
volume micropipette aspiration serves only to demonstrate
comparative behavior of the membrane and substructures, and
these deformation experiments cannot be interpreted in terms of

the models from which intrinsic membrane material properties
have been determined in erythrocyte membranes (6.7). Large
deformations presumably induce large tensions in the membranes
as surface redundancies are smoothed, thus limiting
interpretations. The relative information presented for small
deformations shows the leukocytes resistance to surface
deformation to be five to eight times that of normal
erythrocytes, however this comparison should be viewed with
caution since significant tension may exist in the case of the
leukocytes. It is notable that the lymphocyte may be somewhat
less 'deformable' than the granulocyte, and that both the
lymphocyte from chronic lymphocytic leukemia (CLL) and the
lymphoblast behave like the normal human lymphocyte. Similarly
the granulocyte from chronic myelocyte leukemia resembles the
neutrophilic granulocyte but the myeloblast from AML is more
resistant to small surface deformation than the normal
granulocyte, in keeping with earlier observations of cellular
deformability of myeloblasts (12).

Table 2
Temperature effect on recovery time in leukocytes

Cell type	Recovery time, T_c Seconds		
	20 °C	25 °C	37 °C
Control erythrocyte	0.17	0.13	0.07
Lymphocyte		0.9 - 11.6	0.8 - 5.3
Granulocyte		0.37	.31

Minimal effects of raising the temperature to 37°C were
observed despite detectable increase in granulocyte diameter
7.1 to 7.3 μm which might be expected to result in reduced
cytoplasmic resistance. This contrasts with the significant
change in elastic shear modulus of normal erythrocyte membranes
and the approximately three fold reduction in surface viscosity
of erythrocyte membrane as temperature is raised from 20 to
37°C (11).

Studies of whole cell deformation were unsuccessful for granulocytes at 25 and 37°C due to cell adherence to the glass pipette despite coating glass surfaces with fibrinogen or plasma. Lymphocyte whole cell deformation was accomplished in micropipettes having internal diameters ranging from 2.6 to 3.6 μ:

Table 3

Entrance of lymphocytes in glass micropipettes

Channel diameter, μ	ΔP dynes/cm^2	% Cells entering	T, seconds
2.6	5000	70	94 ± 57
2.8	5000	81	43 ± 26
3.6	3000	100	26 ± 15

The limiting factor was the relatively undeformable nucleus which constitutes approximately one half the volume of the lymphocyte.

Flow channel experiments. Figure 1 indicates the relative extension of normal lymphocytes and cells from patients having CLL or ALL. It is important to recognize the geometrical differences among cells and in the normal vs patient cell populations have an effect on the assumptions concerning fluid drag force on the cells ($F \approx \tau_w \cdot A_p$, where τ_w = shear stress at the chamber surface and A_p = projected area of the cell). However the data are remarkably similar in distribution and regressions.

Figure 1

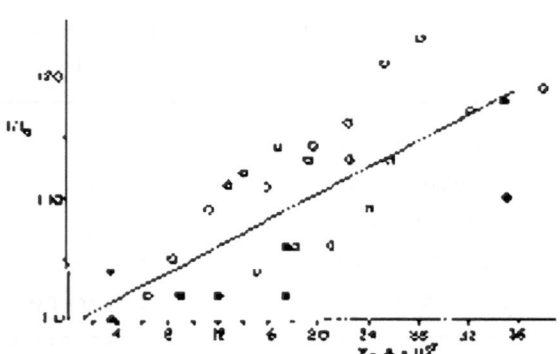

Extension, l of lymphocytes vs wall shear stress τ_w x projected area A_p in a flow channel. l_o = initial cell length. Normal cells = ___; lymphocytes in chronic leukemia = ·; lymphoblasts in acute leukemia = o.

Detachment of leukocytes from plasma-coated glass
and from endothelial cells. Erythrocytes detached from a
figrinogen-coated surface at the force of gravity (13) i.e. a
force/cell of 10^{-8} dynes or for a projected cell area of 50
μm^2, a shear stress of 0.02 dynes/cm^2.

Table 4

Detachment of leukocytes from glass & endothelial cell surfaces

Cell type	Minimum stress for detachment, dyn/cm^2	
	from plasma/glass	from endothelial cell
Lymphocyte	1.8	0.2
Granulocyte	4.6 - 11.3	4.8 - ↑
Erythrocyte	2.1	0.05

Lymphocytes resembled erythrocytes in these experiments, with
little tendency to adhere to endothelial cells; occasional
exceptions, < 1%, were considered to be damaged cells. In
contrast, as shown in Table 4, granulocytes require
considerably more force for detachment from plasma-coated glass
surface of the flow channels or from cultured endothelial cells
in monolayer over the flow channel surface.

Flow channel experiments were corraborated by aspiration of
adherent lymphocytes and granulocytes in a 4.0 μm micropipette
which had been coated with fibrinogen to reduce granulocyte
adhesion. In the case of granulocytes a small number of
neutrophiles adhered to endothelial cells at stresses greater
than 100 dynes/cm^2.

4. DISCUSSION

Many observations of blood cells in microvessels have led
to qualitative descriptions of leukocyte behavior and the
conclusions that granulocytes and lymphocytes are relatively
rigid (14,15). Because leukocytes are spherical in shape and
have a great excess of membrane it has been impossible to
define precisely intrinsic membrane properties and until the
present theoretical work of Skalak, Chien, Schmid-Schonbein and

co-workers little effort to develop adequate models for
leukocytes has been made. The present studies, with the
caveats concerning techniques emphasize the behavior of
leukocytes as spherical bodies relatively less deformable than
normal erythrocytes. Lymphocytes appear to be more rigid than
granulocytes and as observed earlier (4,12) blastic precursors
of granulocytes are less deformable than corresponding mature
forms, whereas the granulocytes in chronic myelocytic leukemia
and lymphocytes in chronic lymphocytic leukemia resemble their
normal counterparts. Little temperature effect was noted in
these experiments in which motility is inhibited although
granulocytes tend to be somewhat more deformable at 37°.
Ultimately, it will be important to define properties of
actively metabolizing granulocytes capable of motility and
phagocytosis, to appreciate their contribution to rheology of
the microcirculation.

Recovery time, as an estimate of the viscous behavior of
leukocytes is limited in interpretability since relative
contributions of cytoplasm, membrane and cytostructure cannot
be defined. The data of Table 2 suggest considerable
variability in the population of lymphocytes, particularly
since a potential variable, duration of deformation, was
constant. On this basis alone lymphocytes might be anticipated
to exert greater influence than granulocytes in the
capillaries, however, observations in vivo (1,3) indicate the
importance of the granulocyte in obstruction. The high minimum
stress for granulocyte detachment from both plasma-coated glass
and the endothelial cell surface implies that adhesion, in
addition to the relatively rigid nuclear lobes, may result in
its observed behavior. The entrance of both granulocytes and
lymphocytes in fibrinogen-coated large micropipettes of
diameters similar to small capillaries suggests that adhesion
to capillary endothelium and not simply the cells' rheologic
properties is important to their influence on the
microcirculation.

ACKNOWLEDGMENT
This paper is based on work partially supported by U.S. National Institutes of Health Grants HL 18208, HL 16421, and Contract No. DE-ACO2-76EV03490 with the U.S. Department of Energy at the University of Rochester Department of Radiation Biology and Biophysics and has been assigned Report No. UR-3490-2071.

REFERENCES
1. Bagge U, Brånemark PI. 1978. White blood cell rheology. An intravital study in man. Adv. Microcirc. 7: 1-17.
2. Schmid-Schönbein GW, Skalak R, Usami S, Chien S. 1980. The interaction of red and white blood cells in capillary and postcapillary blood vessels. Microvasc. Res. 19: 45-70.
3. Olofsson J, Bagge U, Brånemark PI. 1972. Influence of white blood cells on the distribution of blood in microvascular compartments. Bibl. anat. 11: 405-410.
4. Lichtman MA. 1973. Rheology of leukocytes, leukocyte suspensions and blood in leukemia. J. Clin. Invest. 52: 350.
5. Hochmuth RM, Mohandas N, Spaeth EE, Williamson JR, Blackshear PL, Johnson DW. 1972. Surface adhesion, deformation and detachment at low shear of red cells and white cells. Trans Amer Soc Art Int Organs Trans XVIII: 325-334.
6. Evans EA, La Celle PL. 1975. Intrinsic material properties of the erythrocyte membrane indicated by mechanical analysis of deformation. Blood 45: 29-43.
7. Hochmuth RM, Worthy PR, Evans EA. 1979. Red cell extensional recovery and the determination of membrane viscosity. Biophys. J. 26: 101-114.
8. Waugh RE, La Celle PL. 1980. Abnormalities in the membrane material properties of hereditary spherocytes. Biomech. Engineering 102: 240-246.
9. Evans EA. 1973. New membrane concept applied to the analysis of fluid shear and micropipette-deformed red blood cells. Biophys. J. 13: 941-954.
10. Chien S, Sung KLP, Skalak R, Usami S. 1978. Theoretical and experimental studies on viscoelastic properties of erythrocyte membrane. Biophys. J. 24: 463-487.
11. Hochmuth RM, Buxbaum KL, Evans EA. 1980. Temperature dependence of the viscoelastic recovery of red cell membrane. Biophys. J. 29: 177-182.
12. Lichtman MA. 1970. Cellular deformability during maturation of the myeloblast. Possible role in marrow egress. N. Engl. J. Med. 283: 943.
13. Ponder E. 1965. The stickiness of red cells and ghosts. In: Biophysical Mechanisms in Vascular Homeostasis and Intravascular Thrombosis. Ed. N. Sawyer, Appleton Century-Crofts, New York, p.53.
14. Clark ER, Clark EL. 1935. Observations on changes in blood vascular endothelium in the living animal. Amer. J. Anat. 57: 385-438.
15. Brånemark PI. 1964. Intracapillary behavior of the blood. Bibl anat 4: 491-495.

RHEOLOGY OF LEUKOCYTE SUSPENSIONS

GILES R.COKELET and MARSHALL A. LICHTMAN

INTRODUCTION

Very high concentrations of leukocytes in blood are detrimental to the circulation because of microvascular occlusion, as described, for example, by U. Bagge (1). They could also be detrimental because, since the leukocytes are relatively undeformable particles, high concentrations of leukocytes could cause blood viscosity to be abnormally high, leading to an increased heart-work requirement. However, leukemic patients, while having high leukocrits, generally have low erythrocrits, the erythrocrit falling slightly faster with increasing leukocrit than what is needed to keep the total cytocrit constant (2). Because of this tendency to have a more or less constant total cytocrit, the influences of erythrocytes and leukocytes on the viscosity of the bloods from patients tend to counterbalance each other. The relationship between leukocrit and viscosity for bloods from patients has not been clearly established, some literature reports indicating slightly higher viscosities for leukemic bloods compared to normal blood of the same total cytocrit (2) and other reports indicating no relation-ship between viscosity and leukocrit (3).

Because patients with high leukocrits are often anemic, those who have had very high leukocrits reduced by leukophoresis might be considered as possible recipients of packed red cells, to relieve the effects of their anemia. The question is then one of how many red cells they can receive. Because of this question, we began to look into the rheology of red blood cell (RBC) - white blood cell (WBC) mixtures suspended in blood plasma.

This is to be considered a preliminary report of our research on this subject, because of the limited number of observations

which we have, and because of the presence of several as yet
incompletely investigated questions about such matters as the
effect of leukocyte type on blood viscosity and the effects (if
any) of suspension pretreatment, time, etc. on the suspension
properties. Nevertheless, some general observations seem apparent
at this time, and these are presented.

METHODS

White cell rich blood cell suspensions were obtained from
two sources: (1) as blood samples from leukemic patients, and
(2) as white cell concentrates obtained by sedimentation techniques from leukaphoresis residue packs. Red cells and plasma
from normal subjects with the same blood type as the source of
the WBC were used to prepare mixtures of WBC and RBC in plasma.
EDTA was used as the anticoagulant.

The total packed cell volume of the suspensions ("apparent
cytocrit", C_a) was determined by centrifugation of suspensions
in microhematocrit tubes at about 10,000xg for 7 minutes. In
general, the WBC pack and RBC pack were clearly separated, so
that the "apparent leukocrit", L_a, and "apparent erythrocrit",
H_a, could be determined. The packing factor for the red cell
pack was taken as 0.98 and that for the leukocyte pack was taken
as 0.81 (4). Use of these packing factors permits calculation
of the "true total cell volume fraction", C_r, and the "true" WBC
and RBC volume fractions, L_r and H_r.

Cell suspensions were also diluted with isotonic saline (by
a weighing method) and the cells in the diluted suspensions were
counted and sized with a Celloscope electronic particle analyzer.
The erythrocyte electronic shape factor was taken to be 1.04 and
the leukocyte electronic shape factor was taken as 1.38 (4).
These data were used to calculate L_r and H_r of the original
suspension; using the packing factors cited above, L_a, H_a, and
C_a could be calculated and compared with the values obtained by
the microhematocrit tube method. The values of the real cytocrit,
calculated by the two methods, usually differed by less than 5%
of their mean.

Rheological properties of suspensions were measured at $37^{\circ}C$

with two viscometers: a modified GDM concentric-cylinder viscometer for shear rates between 0.1 and 55 sec^{-1}, and a Wells-
Brookfield cone-and-plate viscometer for shear rates between 150
and 1500 sec^{-1}.

RESULTS AND DISCUSSION

    Typical data for WBC-RBC mixtures suspended in plasma are
shown in Figure 1, along with data for RBC suspended in the same
plasma. For all these suspensions, the apparent cytocrit, C_a,
has been made equal to 0.44. At high shear rates, the WBC-rich
suspensions are much more viscous than the blood, due to differences in cellular deformability, but at very low shear rates the
blood is much more viscous, due to differences in cellular
aggregability. The WBC-rich suspensions show the rheological
behavior of suspensions of non-aggregating particles which are
slightly deformable, but in this case the lymphocytes may not be
deformable in a whole cell sense; perhaps only its surface

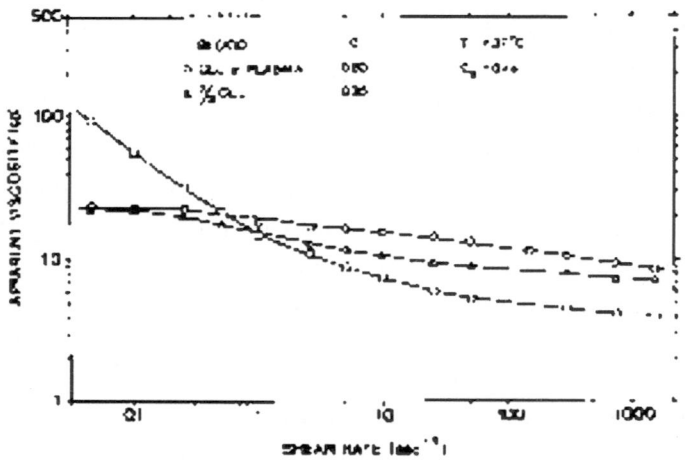

Figure 1. Typical apparent viscosity data, as a function of
shear rate, for two WBC-RBC mixtures in normal plasma, and for
blood. All suspensions have the same apparent total cytocrit of
0.44. The number fraction of all cells which are WBC is given
after the suspension name in the legend.

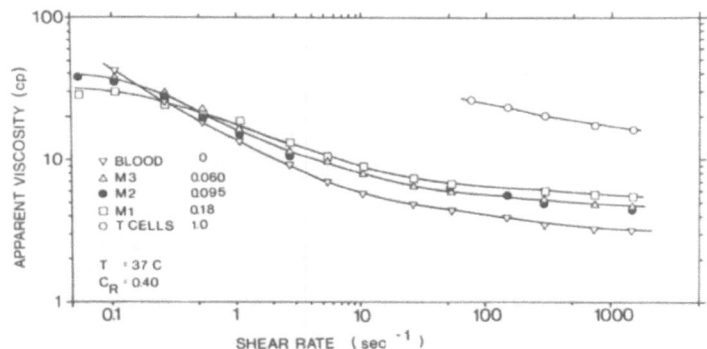

Figure 2. Apparent viscosity versus shear rate for five WBC-RBC mixtures suspended in normal plasma; all suspensions have a real total cytocrit of 0.40. The number fraction of all cells which are WBC is given after the suspension name. The data for M2 and M3 were almost identical; if no symbol for M2 is shown at a shear rate, that datum is the same as that for M3.

"roughness" changes with change in shear stress so that inter-particle exchange of momentum is more efficient at low shear rates.

It must be noted that these suspensions do not have equal true cytocrits, C_r. If data are obtained for WBC-RBC mixtures in plasma at equal real cytocrits, C_r, the data appear as in Figure 2. Now the blood appears to have lower apparent viscosities at given shear rates than in Figure 1, but this is because in Figure 1 the blood C_r was larger than the C_r values for the WBC-RBC mixtures, while in Figure 2 the C_r values are all the same. Other more subtle differences exist between these two figures, but the general rheological features remain the same.

The effect of cellular composition on the suspension rheological properties is more easily seen in the cross-plots of these data, shown in Figure 3. Starting with the panel for a shear rate of 1500 sec^{-1}, it is seen that this plot of apparent viscosity versus the number fraction of all cells which are WBC (C_r held constant) is linear over the entire composition range; replacing WBC with an equal volume of RBC always results in a lower apparent viscosity. It would be expected that this plot, if made at constant apparent total cytocrit, C_a, would have a lower

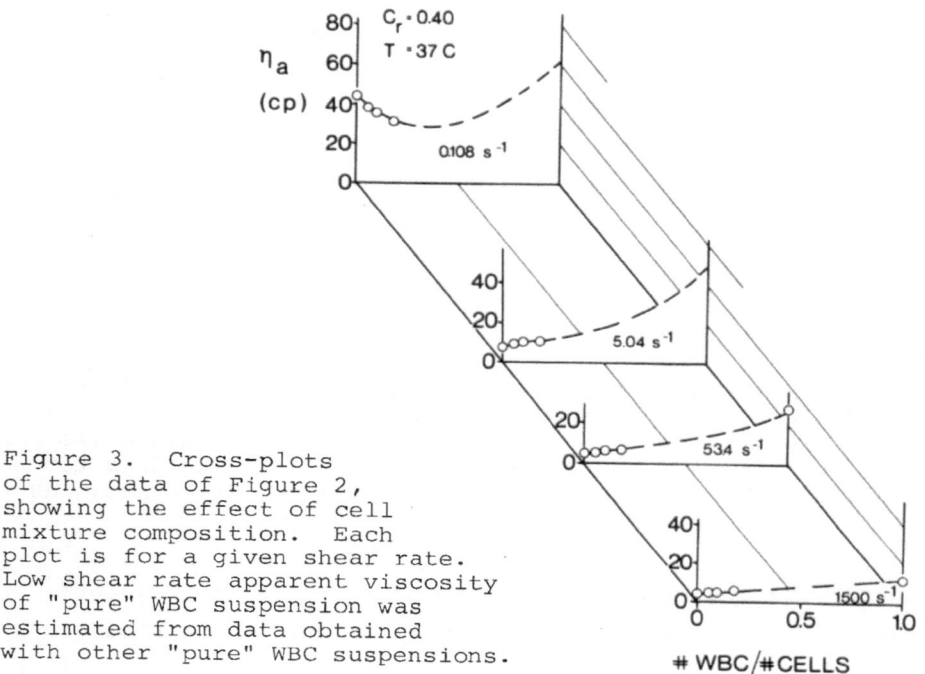

Figure 3. Cross-plots
of the data of Figure 2,
showing the effect of cell
mixture composition. Each
plot is for a given shear rate.
Low shear rate apparent viscosity
of "pure" WBC suspension was
estimated from data obtained
with other "pure" WBC suspensions.

slope to the curve.

The general behavior shown in this very high shear rate
panel continues as the shear rate is lowered, although the
curve begins to show nonlinearities. At very low shear rates,
such as 0.108 sec^{-1}, shown in the upper panel, the curve shows a
minimum so that some WBC-RBC mixtures have lower apparent viscosities than suspensions much richer in either WBC or RBC.

The data shown in this figure are obviously not sufficient
in number. Data from all our tests and literature data can be
combined, but before considering one such composite graph, a
few comments about the literature data may be useful. Two earlier
studies, by Steinman and Charm (3) and Lichtman (2) determined
the shear stress - shear rate data for blood cell suspensions
and then fitted the data with the Casson equation, which is a
linear relationship between the square root of the shear stress

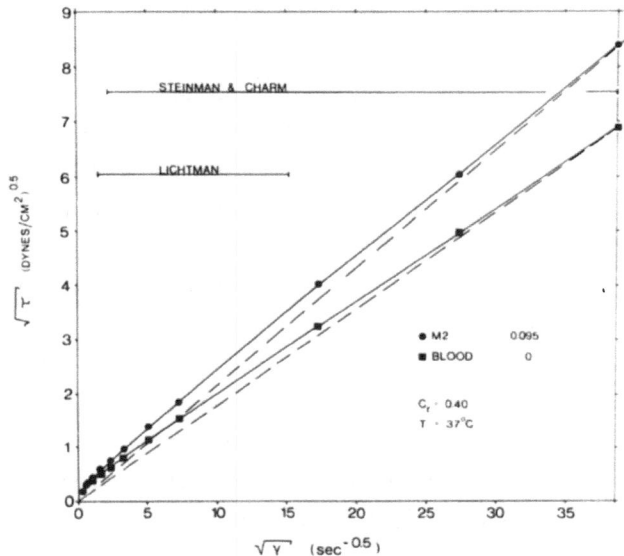

Figure 4. A "Casson plot" of the square root of the shear stress versus the square root of the shear rate, data for blood and suspension M2 of Figure 2. The shear rate ranges used by Lichtman and Steinman and Charm are indicated by the horizontal bars.

and the square root of the shear rate. The square of the slope of this plot was reported as the "minimum apparent viscosity" - which it would be if the data were fitted by such a relationship over the entire shear rate range.

Figure 4 shows such a "Casson plot" of the data for the blood and one of the WBC-RBC mixtures shown in Figure 2. A number of observations can be made from this plot:

(a) The data for neither suspension fit a straight line over the entire range of shear rates; the Casson equation does not represent the data over the shear rate range.

(b) The ranges of shear rates used by Steinman and Charm, and by Lichtman are indicated. The data for a suspension in each of these shear rate ranges could be fit with a straight line, but the slope of the fitted line would be lower for the Steinman-Charm data than for the Lichtman data.

(c) The actual high shear rate Newtonian viscosity is given by the square of the slope of the line from the origin of this

52

plot to the data at very high shear rates; such a line is approximated by the dashed line in each case. From this plot, it
appears that the minimum apparent viscosities reported by
Steinman and Charm underestimate the high shear rate apparent
viscosities, while the minimum apparent viscosities reported by
Lichtman are approximately correct because in the shear rate
range of his data the Casson equation slope is close to the slope
of the Newtonian viscosity line to the high shear rate data.
With these comments as background, let us now consider the data
shown in Figure 5.

Figure 5 shows high shear rate data for WBC-RBC mixtures
suspended in plasma or isotonic saline (Steinman and Charm data).
The real total cytocrit, C_r, is held constant at 0.40. The data
are plotted as relative viscosity, or reported minimum apparent
viscosity divided by the suspending medium viscosity, versus the
fraction of the total cell volume which is WBC volume - effectively, since the total real cytocrit is constant, the abscissa is
proportional to the real leukocrit, L_r. The two unfilled symbols
represent data for suspensions with total cytocrits of 0.37

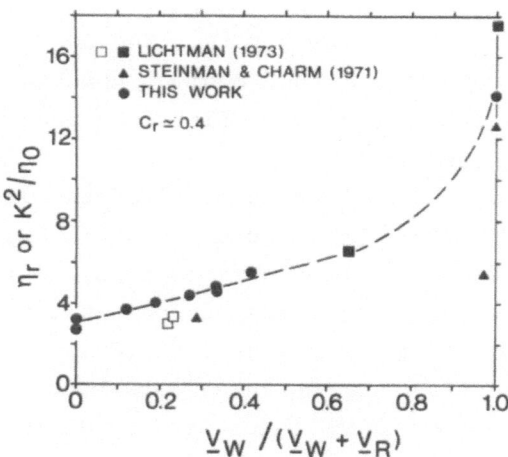

Figure 5. The high shear rate (1500 sec^{-1}) relative apparent
viscosity or (for the literature data) the "minimum apparent
viscosity" divided by the suspending medium viscosity versus the
fraction of the total cell volume which is WBC volume. The real
total cytocrit is constant at 0.40. The two open squares represent data for suspensions with real total cytocrits of 0.37.

instead of 0.40, and as expected are below the curve. Also, as expected from the comments made about Figure 4, the data of Steinman and Charm are below the curve. The data for "pure" leukocyte suspensions are scattered, reflecting experimental difficulties as well perhaps as potential problems arising from preparative handling of cells, etc. These data are all for lymphocytes. In calculating compositions for the literature data, it was assumed that the literature compositions were based on packed cell volumes and that the packing factors were the same as used in our calculations.

The linearity shown by the curve in Figure 5, up to WBC cellular volume fractions of about 0.7, is striking, as is the sharp increase in relative viscosity with increasing WBC concentration above this critical concentration. This critical concentration corresponds to a real leukocrit of about 0.3.

Another collection of data, for "pure" leukocyte suspensions, is shown in Figure 6. The ordinate of this plot is the same as in Figure 5, but on the abscissa are plotted the real and the

Figure 6. High shear rate data for "pure" lymphocyte suspensions. The abscissa is the real leukocrit (filled symbols) and the apparent leukocrit (open symbols). The compositions reported in the literature are indicated by the open symbols; the filled symbol connected to the unfilled symbol shows the composition calculated by assuming a WBC packing factor of 0.81. The curve is for suspensions of rigid, smooth spheres.

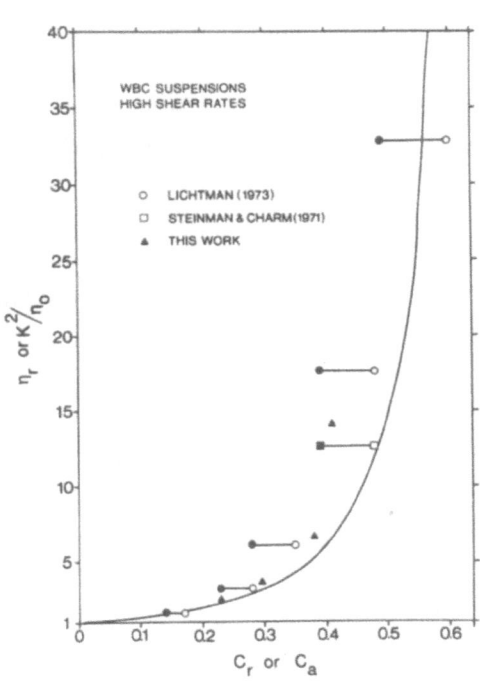

apparent cytocrit. These data are for high shear rates (subject to earlier comments on reported minimum apparent viscosities), and the literature data are plotted both with the reported ("apparent") cytocrit, C_a, and the calculated "real" cytocrit, C_r. The curve represents the experimental data for suspensions of rigid spheres, as reviewed by Rutgers (5).

It is not clear how one should draw the curve to represent these data, but for C_r above about 0.25 - 0.30, the relative viscosities are greater than those shown by comparable suspensions of rigid, smooth spheres. If the data for lower shear rates were plotted here, the relative viscosities of the leukocyte suspensions, especially above C_r of about 0.25-0.30, would deviate even further from the rigid, smooth sphere suspensions curve. Three comments can be made relative to this plot:

(a) The fact that the data are above the smooth hard sphere curve implies that these WBC suspensions are more efficient at transferring momentum between adjacent layers of suspension than suspensions of rigid smooth spheres. This may reflect additional effectiveness due to the "roughness" of the WBC surface, which increases as the shear rate decreases, and

(b) The fact that the suspensions are non-Newtonian, with higher apparent viscosities atlower shear rates, is compatible with either a slightly deformable particle or a rough particle whose roughness increases as shear rate decreases, or both. Time-dependent behavior of WBC-rich suspensions has not been observed, on the time scale needed to deform leukocytes, and it is therefore speculated that the non-Newtonian behavior of these suspensions is primarily due to changes in cell surface "roughness".

(c) While a critical concentration is not as well defined here as in the previous figure, there does seem to be one at about C_r of 0.25-0.30. Lichtman, from a semi-log plot of his data, found a critical leukocrit at about 0.20. This poorly defined critical lymphocyte concentration corresponds in a model of uniformly spaced lymphocytes to a spherical particle with a diameter of 7.4 microns (for the WBC) in each cubic volume element representing suspension volume, with each cubic volume

element having an edge length of about 9 microns.
These limited data indicate, as a first approximation, that
this critical WBC concentration is not very sensitive to the RBC
concentration.

SUMMARY

The rheological properties of suspensions of WBC-RBC mixtures
in normal plasma can be summarized as follows:

(1) Bloods which are very rich in WBC are non-Newtonian, but
tend towards Newtonian behavior at very low shear rates (e.g.,
$0.1 \sec^{-1}$) and above about $1500 \sec^{-1}$. This behavior is consistent
with a model of these suspensions which consists of deformable,
aggregatable particles (RBC), and nonaggregatable particles (WBC)
which are essentially undeformable and whose surface is rough, the
nature of this roughness changing with the level of the shear
stress.

(2) At high and moderate shear rates, when the total cell
volume concentration is held constant, the relationship between
suspension apparent viscosity and the number fraction of all cells
which are leukocytes is essentially linear, with viscosity increasing with leukocyte concentration. At very low shear rates, this
relationship becomes nonlinear with a minimum viscosity appearing
at a leukocyte fraction between zero and unity.

(3) When expressed in terms of the leukocrit, the suspension apparent viscosity, under a condition of constant total cell
volume fraction, is a linear function of leukocrit up to a critical leukocrit of about 0.25-0.30; this relationship has a relatively small slope. Above the critical leukocrit, viscosity begins to
increase rapidly with increase in leukocrit.

ACKNOWLEDGEMENTS

The experimental work was performed partly under Contract No.
DE-ACO2-76EVO3490 with the U. S. Dept. of Energy at the University
of Rochester Department of Radiation Biology and Biophysics and
has been assigned Report No. UR-3490-2091, and partly with support
from NIH Grants HL-18208 and HL-23355. This report was prepared
while the first author was the recipient of a U. S. Senior Scien-

56

tist Award from the Alexander von Humboldt-Stiftung and resident
at the Institut für normale und pathologishe Physiologie der
Universität zu Köln, West Germany. Professor Gaehtgens, Frau L.
Glahe and Frau K. Klein are thanked for their assistance in
preparing this report.

REFERENCES
(1)   Bagge, U., this conference.
(2)   Lichtman, M., J. Clin. Invest., $\underline{52}$. 350-358 (1973).
(3)   Steinman, M. H. and S. E. Charm, Blood, $\underline{38(3)}$, 299-301 (1971)
(4)   Segel, G. B., G. R. Cokelet and M. A. Lichtman, Blood,
       $\underline{57(5)}$, 894-899 (1981).
(5)   Rutgers, I. R., Rheol. Acta, $\underline{2}$, 305 (1962).

RHEOLOGICAL MECHANISMS CONTRIBUTING TO WBC-MARGINATION

U. NOBIS, A. R. PRIES and P. GAEHTGENS

Since the function of WBC is mainly fullfilled in the extra-vascular tissue, these cells have to emigrate from the circulation which is only used as a transport system. Before active emigration can take place the leukocytes must be in a position where they can interact with the endothelium through which they penetrate. This interaction can only be established if the WBC travel close to the vessel wall. Therefore the phenomenon of margination must be considered as a first step in the series of events constituting leukocyte extravasation. Since active locomotion of WBC within the flowing blood is impossible, leukocytes must be passively displaced towards the endothelial surface. This displacement can be favored or inhibited by the hydrodynamic and rheological flow conditions (1). Even if the mechanism of WBC-margination and the following steps leading to emigration are not yet fully understood, it is well known that these phenomena occur mainly in the small venules of the microcirculation (2, 8).

It has been suggested that upon leaving the venous end of a capillary the WBC are pushed towards the vessel wall by RBC passing them (6). According to our own observations (3) this takes place only if the leukocytes occupy between 50-80% of the vessel diameter, so that they act as an obstacle to the free flow of the erythrocytes. It is difficult to believe that WBC-displacement due to RBC-overtaking alone would be sufficient to account for leukocyte margination in larger venules and the enhancement of margination in inflammation and so-called low flow states. Therefore we studied the rheological factors determining the radial distribution of WBC in flow. This was done in blood-perfused glass capillaries in which WBC-adhesion did not occur.

58

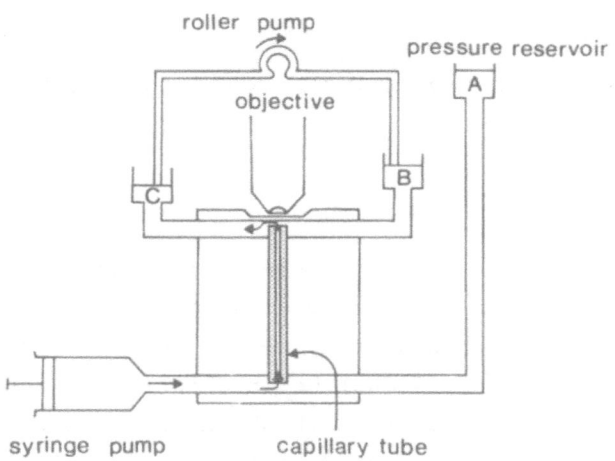

FIGURE 1. Schematic drawing of the experimental set-up

Fig. 1 shows a schematic diagram of the experimental set-up.
Glass capillaries (I.D. 34-69 µm, length 3.6 cm) were mounted
vertically on the stage of a fluorescence microscope. Blood was
delivered by a syringe pump into the tubing connected to the
pressure reservoir A. Because of the applied hydrostatic head,
some fraction of this blood flowed upward through the capillary
tube. The driving pressure across the capillary was changed by
varying the height of the reservoir A. Blood flowing out of the
upper end of the tube was removed by a constant cross-flow of
saline between the reservoirs B and C.

In order to obtain a distribution of WBC across the tube
diameter which was unaffected by exit effects or the cross-flow,
the objective was focussed 30 µm into the outflow end of the
capillary. The WBC were visualized by the fluorocrome acridine-
orange (10 mg/l blood), and their passage through the focal plane
of the objective was recorded by a television camera on a video-
tape recorder. The experiments were performed with human blood,
anticoagulated with EDTA at a hematocrit of 0.45; the WBC-concentration ranged between 5000-6000/µl.

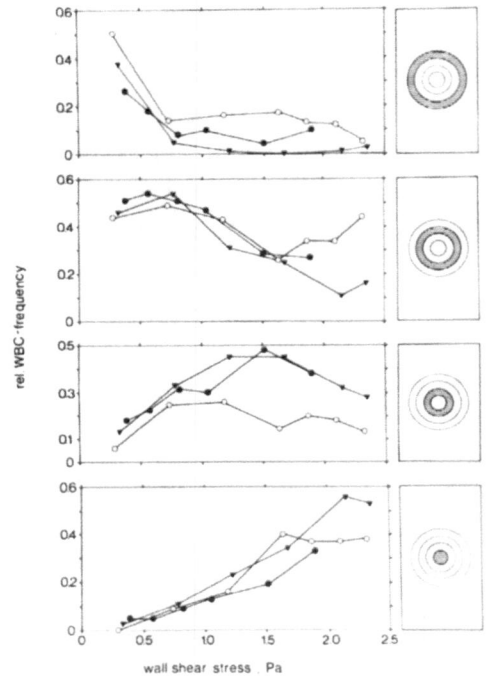

FIGURE 2. Number of WBC in one of four concentric rings (schematically shown on the right) relative to the total number of WBC (relative WBC-frequency) as a function of wall shear stress. Data from three experiments in a 69 μm tube with blood cells suspended in their native plasma.

Fig. 2 shows the results of three experiments in which native blood (i.e. blood cells suspended in their plasma) was used. The number of leukocytes observed in one of four rings relative to the total number of WBC seen (relative frequency) is plotted in each panel as a function of the tube wall shear stress. Each panel summarizes the data obtained in one of the rings of the tube cross section, which is indicated schematically.

At low wall shear stress the maximum frequency of WBC-appearance is in the outermost region of the flow. As the shear stresses are increased, the WBC are redistributed through the intermediate concentric rings towards the centerstream. This finding is consistent with earlier results obtained in vivo (5) and with the conclusion that "the slowing of the blood stream......would

make it easier for the leukocytes to accumulate close to the
vessel wall" (1).

In order to test whether the observed shear-dependent WBC-
redistribution is a consequence of shear-dependent RBC flow
behaviour, the plasma of the blood was replaced by either high
molecular weight dextran solution or saline, thereby modifying
the aggregation tendency of the red blood cells.

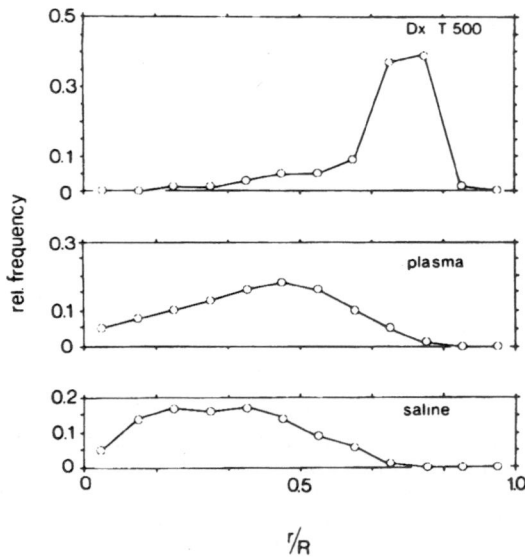

FIGURE 3. Relative frequency of WBC plotted versus radial distance
from the tube center (r/R) for blood cells suspended in 1% dextra
solution (Dx T500), plasma and saline. Tube diameter 69 μm.

Fig. 3 shows results obtained in a 69 μm tube at a wall shear
stress of 1.25 Pa. In this figure, the relative frequency of WBC
is shifted towards the tube wall in the presence of Dx T500 and
towards the tube center if saline is used as suspending medium.

These findings suggest that the radial frequency distribution
of WBC in the flowing blood is not so much a consequence of their
own flow behaviour or flow properties, but much more dependent on
the interaction with the red blood cells surrounding them. In the

presence of high shear stresses and/or the absence of red cell
aggregation (e.g. in saline) the frequency of WBC-appearance is
uniform in the central region of the flow, but leukocytes are
not seen in the high shear region close to the tube wall. On the
other hand, at increased erythrocyte aggregation (in dextran) they
are significantly displaced into the marginal flow regions. If
RBC-aggregation is absent, the leukocytes, being the largest
blood cells, travel in the center of the tube or vessel, while
WBC-displacement occurs if red cell aggregates occupy the centerstream. This observation is in agreement with in vitro results
obtained by PALMER (4) and with the conclusion of VEJLENS that
"larger particles are transported at a greater distance from the
wall of the tube than smaller particles" (7).

The flow conditions in precapillary arterioles are normally
characterized by relatively high shear stresses, whereas the increased total cross-sectional area in the postcapillary venules
leads to significantly lower flow velocities and hence shear
stresses in these vessels. Thus, the described shear-dependent
mechanism of WBC-margination favors the interaction between leukocytes and the vascular endothelium in the postcapillary venules.
Alterations of plasma protein composition which are often seen in
inflammatory diseases likewise favor WBC-margination in venules
as a result of enhanced red cell aggregation tendency.

Interaction between leukocytes and the endothelium can only
occur with those WBC which are found in the outermost fluid layer
of the flowing blood. This is schematically depicted in Fig. 4.
In order to quantitatively evaluate the effectiveness of the
described mechanism of WBC-displacement, an attempt was made to
calculate the fraction (A_F) of the endothelial surface (A_T) at
which this interaction can take place. The parameter A_F is only
a function of leukocyte concentration in the outermost fluid
layer, the width of which was assumed to be equal to the diameter
of a single WBC, i.e. 7 μm. In order to determine the WBC-concentration in this layer (C_{WBC}), the frequency of WBC-appearance
(F_{WBC}) was divided by the cross-sectional area of the peripheral

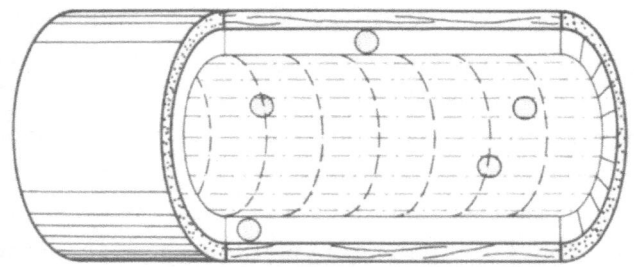

FIGURE 4. Schematic diagram of a vessel section demonstrating
the number of WBC in the marginal fluid layer at any one instant
Only a small fraction of the total endothelial surface is covered
by the WBC in this layer.

sleeve and the mean WBC-velocity v_{WBC} in this sleeve:

$$C_{WBC} = \frac{F_{WBC}}{\pi \cdot (R^2 - r^2) \cdot v_{WBC}}$$

The contact area between a spherical leukocyte in the marginal
layer and the flat endothelial surface is difficult to quantify.
For practical purposes we have assumed a contact area larger than
zero and smaller than the diametrical plane of the WBC. For the
sake of simplicity it is assumed that the fractional area (A_F)
is equal to the fractional volume (V_F) of the marginal sleeve
occupied by the WBC. This is equivalent to representing each WBC
as a cube (with the same volume as the WBC) which has one face in
contact with the endothelial surface:

$$A_F = V_F = \frac{V_{WBC}}{V_T}$$

where V_{WBC} = total volume of all WBC in the marginal layer,
V_T = total volume of the marginal layer.

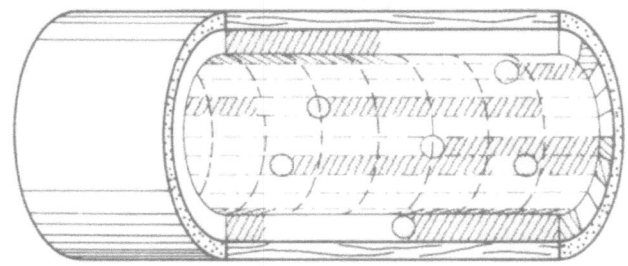

FIGURE 5. Same vessel section as in Fig. 4 after a finite time
interval. The sum of the hatched areas indicates the fraction of
the total endothelial surface which has been "scanned" by the
flowing WBC in the marginal fluid layer.

Furthermore the time Δt required for the total endothelial
surface (A_T) to be "scanned" by the passing leukocytes in the
marginal layer was calculated. Δt is equivalent to the average
time a single endothelial cell has to wait until it is faced by
the next WBC passing over it. This is obviously a function of the
mean velocity of the leukocytes in the marginal layer (v_{WBC}), the
fractional area covered by the WBC at any instant (A_F) and the
dimension of the leukocyte (d, where d = edge length of the cube,
representing the WBC):

$$\Delta t \quad = \quad \frac{1}{A_F} \cdot \frac{1}{v_{WBC}} \cdot d$$

Fig. 5 shows schematically WBC "scanning" the endothelial surface
and aids in understanding the derivation of the above equation.

The above calculations were applied to data obtained in the
presence of Dx T500 and the data obtained with saline as suspending
medium. As shown in Fig. 6, the marginal WBC-concentration in these
two cases is significantly different. The fraction of endothelial
surface covered by leukocytes increases and the time Δt to scan
the total surface area available decreases by a factor of approxi-

64

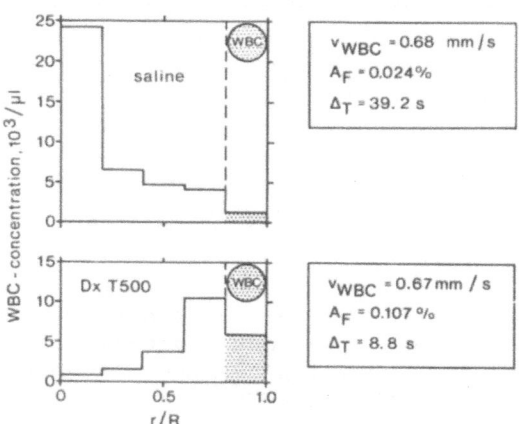

tube diameter 69 μm

$\tau_W : 0.5$ Pa

$v_{WBC} = 0.68$ mm/s
$A_F = 0.024\%$
$\Delta_T = 39.2$ s

$v_{WBC} = 0.67$ mm/s
$A_F = 0.107\%$
$\Delta_T = 8.8$ s

FIGURE 6. The radial distribution of the WBC-concentration obtained in an experiment with saline (top) and Dx T500 (below)
as suspending media. The stippled area represents the WBC-
concentration in the marginal layer whose width is equal to the
diameter of a WBC. On the right the WBC-velocity in the marginal
sleeve (v_{WBC}), the fraction of covered endothelial surface (A_F),
and the time necessary for the total vessel wall to be "scanned"
by passing WBC (Δt) are given.

mately five as a result of the aggregation dependent mechanism
of WBC-displacement.

This analysis cannot describe quantitatively the in vivo
conditions in a system of branching and rejoining microvessels.
It can however serve as an order of magnitude analysis of the
mechanism involved in WBC-margination which eventually leads to
WBC-adhesion. It may be of interest to note that the maximum
possible contact area between leukocytes and the endothelium
(which could be obtained by moving all the WBC in the vessel to
the marginal layer) would amount to only 0.3% of the total
endothelial surface with the leukocyte concentration present in
our experiments. The mechanism described here leads to an A_F of
0.107% (Fig. 6) i.e. approximately 1/3 of the maximum possible,
whereas in the absence of RBC-aggregation less than 1/10 of the
maximum contact area is present.

REFERENCES

1. GRANT, L. (1973) The sticking and emigration of WBC in
      inflammation. The Inflammatory Process 2: 205-249
2. KROGH, A. (1929) The anatomy and physiology of capillaries
      New York, Hafner
3. NOBIS, U., GAEHTGENS, P. (1981) Rheology of WBC during blood
      flow through narrow tubes. Bibl. anat. 20: 211-214
4. PALMER, A. A. (1967) Platelet and leukocyte skimming.
      Bibl. anat. 9: 300-303
5. PHIBBS, R. H. (1966) Distribution of leukocytes in blood
      flowing through arteries. Am. J. Physiol. 210: 919-925
6. SCHMID-SCHÖNBEIN, G. W., USAMI, S., SKALAK, R., CHIEN, S. (1980)
      The interaction of leukocytes and erythrocytes in capillary
      and postcapillary vessels. Microvasc. Res. 14: 45-70
7. VEJLENS, G. (1938) The distribution of leukocytes in the
      vascular system. Acta path. microbiol. scand. 33: 11-239
8. ZWEIFACH, B. W. (1961) Functional behaviour of the micro-
      circulation. Springfield III, Thomas, p. 95

FLOW BEHAVIOR OF WHITE BLOOD CELLS IN VITRO AND IN VIVO
(COMMENTARY)

RICHARD SKALAK

The papers of this Symposium provide sufficient information on the properties of individual WBC, rheology of suspensions containing WBC, and mechanisms of WBC margination to
describe the main features of flow of WBC in venules and
arterioles. The viscoelastic properties of granulocytes and
lymphocytes reported by La Celle et al. and other papers of
this Symposium make it clear that WBC are generally sufficiently stiffer than erythrocytes so that in a suspension of
normal proportions the WBC must behave essentially as rigid
spheres. This is borne out by the bulk rheological measurements of leukocytes suspensions by Cokelet and Lichtman. In
fact in relatively pure leukocyte suspensions the data for
high shear rates shows that the apparent viscosity is higher
for WBC suspensions than for smooth, hard sphere suspensions.
As these authors suggest this probably reflects the effect
of roughness of the WBC surface. By cross-plotting the apparent viscosity for the full range from zero to 100 percent
WBC with a constant total cell volume (erythrocyte volume is
varied to compensate) it is clear that the normal range of
WBC concentrations have very little effect on the bulk viscosity
of blood.

The rheological mechanisms contributing to WBC margination
in a tube 69 µm in diameter reported by Nobis et al. demonstrates
interesting extensions of Fahreus-Lindqvist effects. The
conclusion is that the radial distribution of WBC in flowing
blood is not so much a consequence of their own flow behavior
but is dependent on the interaction with the red blood cells.
In the absence of red cell aggregation the distribution of

WBC is more uniform but near zero close to the tube wall. In the presence of erythrocyte aggregation the WBC are displaced into the marginal flow region. This indicates a mechanism of WBC margination at low flow states when red cell aggregation is to be expected.

In summary in regard to flow in the venules and arterioles the Symposium shows that WBC behave essentially as rigid spheres with little influence on the bulk rheology of blood flow, and with a radial distribution that is determined by interaction with the erythrocytes and/or their aggregates. In low flow states there is clearly sufficient margination of leukocytes to put the burden of whether or not WBC roll or adhere to the endothelium on the surface properties of the WBC and endothelium rather than on the supply side of the WBC flow. The flow properties are interesting but probably not critical in controlling the physiological effects of WBC of interest.

There are nevertheless several points raised by the papers in this Symposium which deserve further exploration. The differences in behavior of granulocytes and lymphocytes cited by La Celle et al., particularly with respect to adhesion to endothelial cells, should be investigated if possible in vivo. The role and properties of endothelium in regard to WBC adhesion needs further exploration. In the future in studying the interaction of the flow properties of WBC and their adhesion or rolling along vessel walls there is a need for the kind of accounting which has been begun in the paper by Nobis et al. Even in the steady flow of blood in a straight tube there is some radial motion and therefore a radial diffusion of WBC in both directions. If there is adhesion, a small diffusion gradient is created. The interplay of delivery of WBC to the wall, its adhesion or rolling, and its eventual release needs to be traced as a transient mass flux and balance so as to account for the number of WBC to be expected under various conditions and the length of time that they may be present. This calls for computations of the diffusion fields and the adhesion characteristics at the same time.

This commentary has been limited primarily to venules and arterioles which are at least two or more times the diameter of the WBC. In smaller vessels, particularly in capillaries, the situation is more complicated and will hopefully be covered in another commentary. Suffice it to say here that in the capillaries the rigidity of the white cell itself can play a role in creating abnormally large resistances and most probably does so in low flow states. Here again the role of the endothelial cell needs more exploration. The possibility of endothelial protrusions or swellings may play a role in impeding WBC in pathological situations. It is also possible that in pathological situations there is some adhesion between the endothelial cell and the WBC. This is a possibility, but not a necessity because of the very stiff nature of the white blood cell and the narrowness of the capillaries. By contrast in the venules and arterioles any rolling or adhesion of WBC must certainly involve a kind of surface bonding of the WBC and the endothelium.

THE ANATOMICAL FEATURES OF LEUKOCYTE EGRESS INTO THE MARROW SINUS

MARSHALL A. LICHTMAN, M.D.

1. INTRODUCTION

Hemopoietic cells proliferate and mature in the intersinal spaces of the marrow. Following maturation the cells enter the circulation through the wall of the marrow sinus. This anatomical process of cell egress has been studied by several laboratories (1-9). In this short review, I will reiterate two features that may be important for the process of marrow egress: 1) the structure of the sinus wall, and 2) the appearance of granulocytes traversing the wall. The process of egress of reticulocytes and megakaryocyte cytoplasm is not relevant to this conference and the reader is referred to previous reports on these matters (1-5,7,8,10,11). Studies also have addressed granulocyte maturation as a prerequisite for egress. Granulocyte deformability, adhesiveness, motility and chemotactic responsiveness are enhanced during maturation and these alterations may facilitate egress (12,13).

2. MARROW SINUS WALL

The marrow sinus wall in rodents, especially the mouse where it has been studied extensively, is composed of a luminal layer of endothelial cells and an abluminal layer of adventitial reticular cells. Between these two cellular layers is an attenuated, interrupted basement lamina (1,3,5,14).

Figure 1 shows the characteristic features of the marrow sinus. The endothelial cell layer is thought to be complete, whereas the adventitial reticular cell layer covers about two-thirds of the abluminal sinus wall in unperturbed animals (10). The endothelium is highly endocytoytic and also contains fenestrae with diaphragms (15). The area of the adventitial cell layer is decreased when erythropoiesis is stimulated by experimental hemolytic anemia, erythropoietin administration or endotoxin administration (2,8,10). This change has been interpreted as one that facilitates egress by reducing the barrier between mature marrow cells and the sinus lumen.

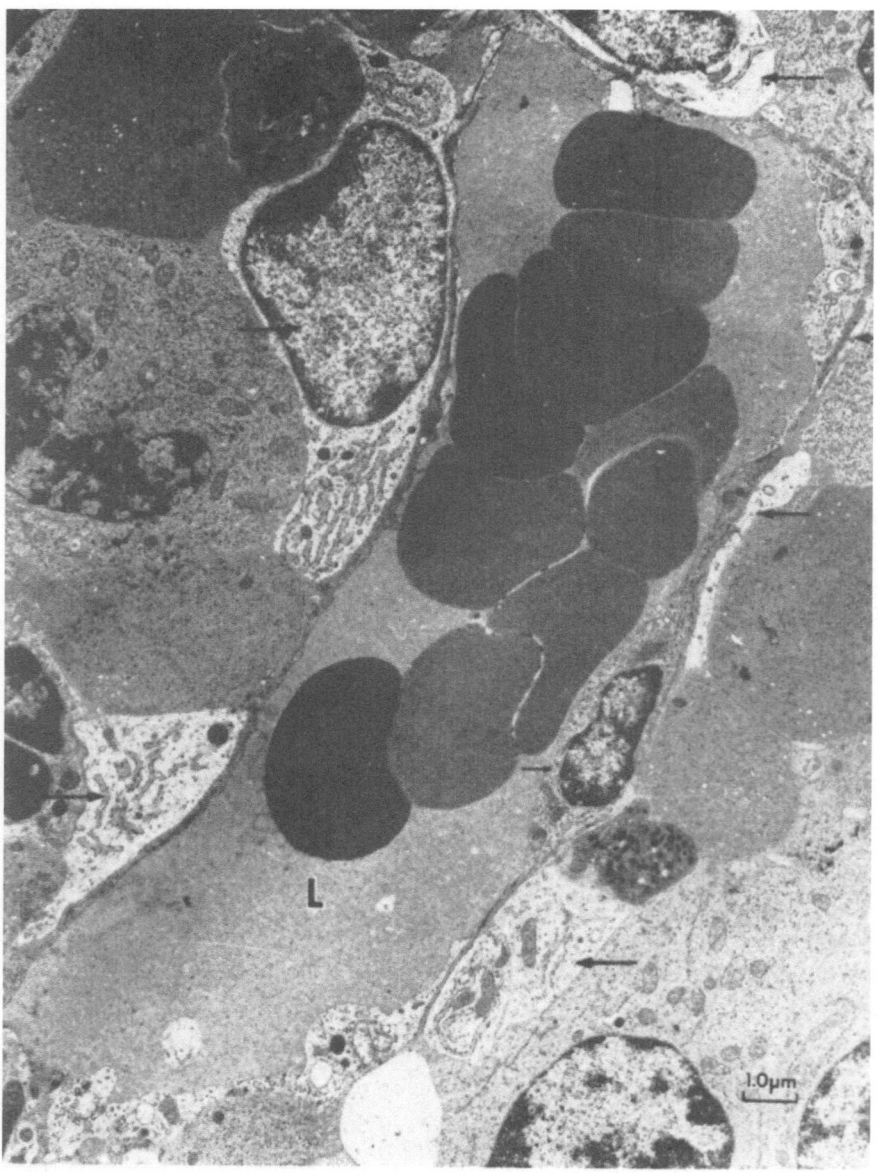

FIGURE 1. TEM of a mouse marrow sinus. The small arrow in the sinus lumen
(L) points to an endothelial cell. The sinus wall is composed of a lumenal
layer of endothelial cells whose cytoplasm can be seen along the circumference
of the sinus lumen. Two adventitial reticular cell bodies are identified
by arrows at the top and upper left of the sinus. The cytoplasm of adventitial reticular cells is discontinuous as it is followed around the
sinus. Four areas of reticular cell cytoplasm are indicated by arrows.

3.   LEUKOCYTES IN EGRESS

Studies have established that cells migrate through an endothelial migration channel as they enter the marrow sinus, rather than between endothelial cells as occurs when neutrophils emigrate from post capillary venules into tissues. The migration channel has a complete covering of endothelial cell membrane, indicating that the leukocyte is in the extra-cellular space as it passes through endothelium and, thus, its passage through the endothelial cell is not a form of emperipolesis. The migration channel is present or develops beside an endothelial cell junction more frequently than is expected by chance (16). Migration pores are thought to develop as the cell penetrates the endothelial cell (16). The chemical basis for the penetration of the endothelial cell by the emigrating leuko-cyte is unknown. Studies of the localization of cationized ferritin in marrow sections have shown that there is a focus of anionic groups on the surface of the migrating cell at the point of contact and penetration of the endothelial cell (17). These anionic groups do not contain n-acetyl neuraminic acid. Although megakaryocyte cytoplasm is often seen producing invaginations of endothelial cells prior to penetration into the sinus, such invaginations are rare when reticulocytes or leukocytes abut the abluminal side of the endothelial cell. Monocytes have been observed invaginating endothelium, however.

During migration the cell undergoes marked deformation as it squeezes through the pore in the endothelial cell. Eosinophils, monocytes and lymphocytes have been observed in egress. Marked deformation of the cell occurs during egress such that the diameter of the migration pore is usually less than one-third the spherical diameter of the cell and occasionally pore diameter may be much less. Nuclear deformation in mononuclear cells occurs during egress. Unlike in vitro studies, using micropipettes, in which nuclei are resistant to extreme deformation, nuclei of cells in egress can be seen to deform markedly.

Leukocytes initiating egress often show a small organelle-poor pseudo-pod extending through the endothelium into the sinus lumen. The appearance of the cell suggests that it is undergoing ameboid movement. The features of leukocyte egress are listed in Table 1.

Figures 2 through 7 show the anatomical features of leukocytes migrating from the hemopoietic spaces into the marrow sinus lumen.

TABLE 1

CHARACTERISTICS OF LEUKOCYTE EGRESS

1. Occurs through a parajunctional transendothelial cell migration pore.

2. Migration pore develops as cell initiates egress.

3. Migration pore is usually short ($<0.6\mu$m) and has an endothelial cell membrane lining.

4. Similar anatomical pattern of egress for neutrophils, eosinophils, monocytes and lymphocytes.

5. Marked cell deformation during egress.

6. Nuclear deformation of mononuclear cells in egress (lymphocytes, monocytes).

7. Apparent ameboid configuration during egress.

8. Polarization of anionic groups on surface of cell in egress at point of endothelial cell contact.

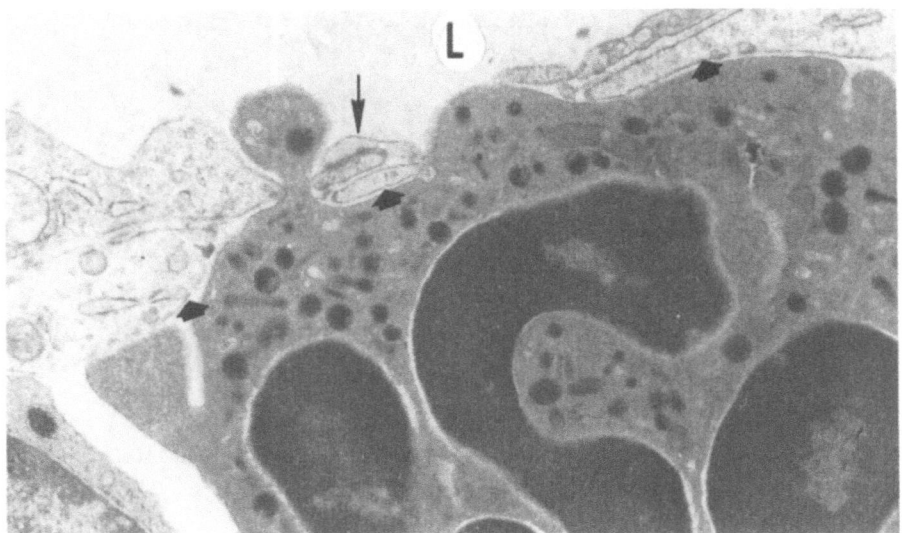

FIGURE 2. Mouse granulocyte penetrating marrow sinus endothelium. An overlapping endothelial cell junction is beneath the long arrow. The marrow sinus lumen is indicated by an "L". The short arrows indicate the cytoplasm of adventitial reticular cells. Two points of penetration by the cell in egress are seen. This dual migration channel is unusual although the pores may be joined at a different level. Note the probing pseudopod on the left is blunted by reticular cell cytoplasm.

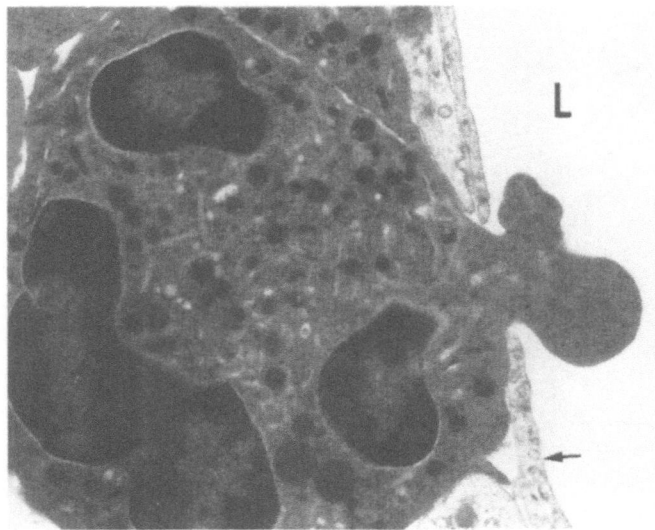

FIGURE 3. Granulocyte pseudopod penetrating mouse marrow sinus endothelium. The lumen is indicated by an "L" and the endothelial cell cytoplasm by the arrow.

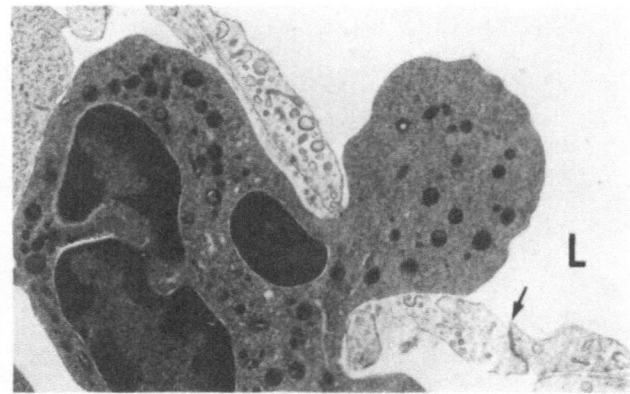

FIGURE 4. Granulocyte penetrating mouse marrow sinus endothelium. An endothelial cell junction is beneath the arrow.

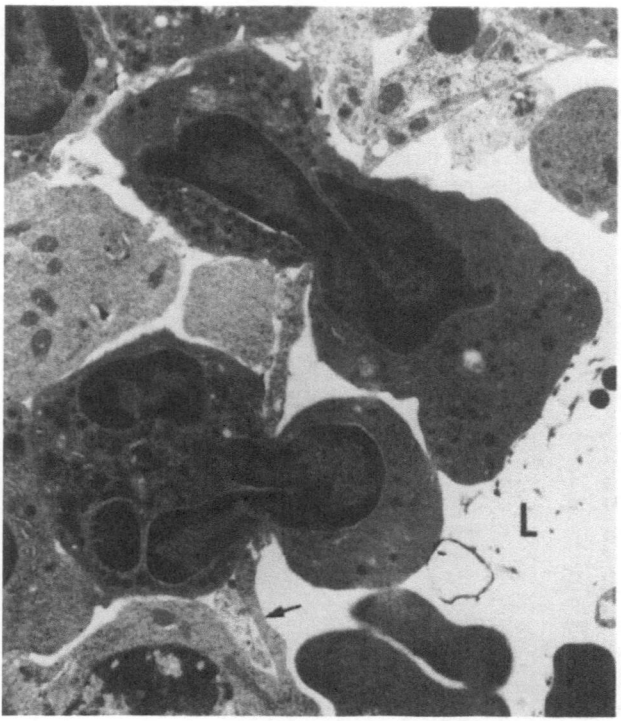

FIGURE 5. Two granulocytes entering a mouse marrow sinus lumen (L). The arrow indicates the endothelial cell cytoplasm. The deformation of the cell is evident as they pass through the endothelial cell cytoplasm.

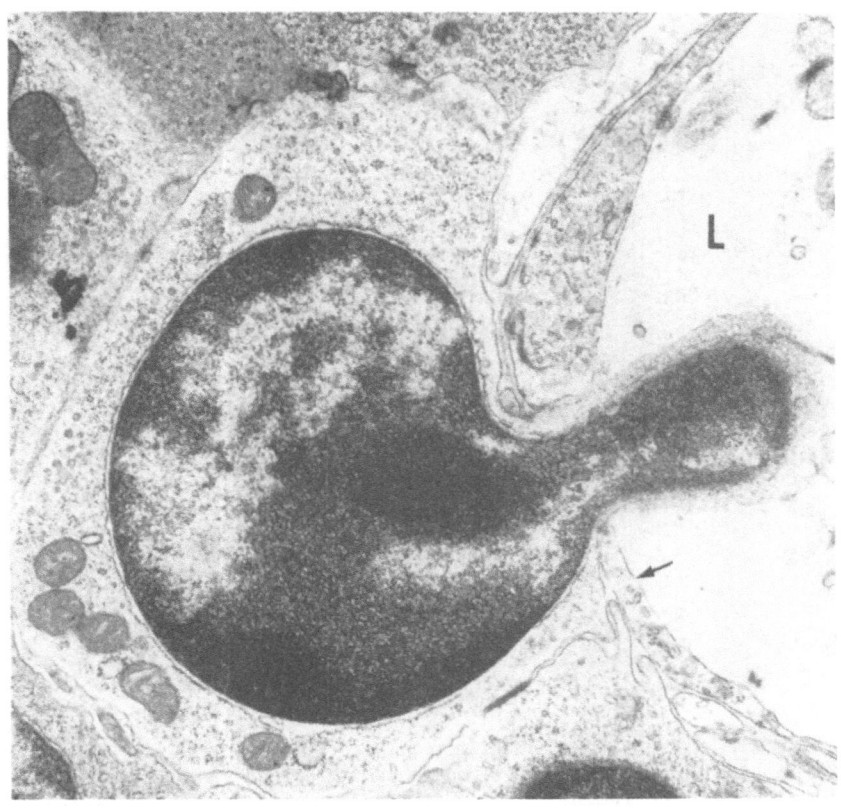

FIGURE 6. Lymphocyte entering a mouse marrow sinus lumen (L). Note the
marked deformation of cell and nucleus. The arrow indicates lumenal
surface of endothelial cell cytoplasm.

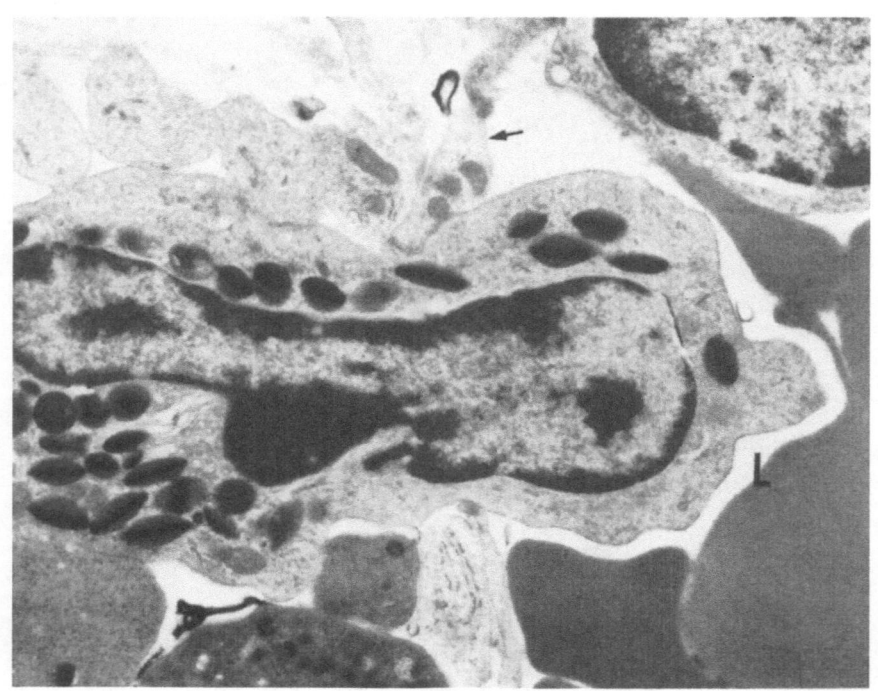

FIGURE 7. Eosinophil entering a mouse marrow sinus lumen (L). The arrow indicates the luminal edge of the endothelial cell cytoplasm.

4. SUMMARY

Although attention has been given to the anatomical process of egress, the biochemical events underlying this process remain to be defined.

5. ACKNOWLEDGEMENT

This report was supported by USPHS Grant HL-18208. Figure 1 is reproduced from Reference 14, and Figures 4, 6 and 7 from Reference 9.

77

REFERENCES

1. Weiss, L. The histopathology of the bone marrow. Clin. Orthop. 52:13, 1967.
2. Weiss, L. Transmural cellular passage in the vascular sinuses of rat bone marrow. Blood. 36:189, 1970.
3. DeBruyn, PPH, Michelson, S., Thomas, TB. The migration of blood cells of the bone marrow through the sinusoidal wall. J. Morphol. 133:417, 1971.
4. DeBruyn, PPH, Michelson, S, Thomas, TB. The migration of blood cells of the bone marrow through the sinus wall. J. Morphol. 133:417, 1971.
5. Campbell, FR. Ultrastructural studies of transmural migration of blood cells in the bone marrow of rats, mice and guinea pigs. Am. J. Anat. 135:521, 1972
6. Weiss, L, Chen, LT. The organization of hemopoietic cords and vascular sinuses in bone marrow. Blood Cells. 1:617, 1975.
7. Becker, RP, DeBruyn, PPH. The transmural passage of blood cells into myeloid sinusoids and the entry of platelets into the sinusoidal circulation. A scanning electron microscopic investigation. Amer. J. Anat. 145:183, 1976.
8. Chamberlain, JK, Leblond, PF, Weed, RI. Reduction of adventitial cell cover: an early direct effect of erythropoietin on bone marrow ultrastructure. Blood Cells. 1:655, 1975.
9. Lichtman, MA, Chamberlain, JK, Santillo, PA. Factors thought to contribute to the regulation of egress of cells from marrow. The Year in Hematology, 1978. p. 243. Edited by Silber, R, LoBue, J and Gordon, AS.
10. Chamberlain, JK, Weiss, L, Weed, RI. Bone marrow sinus cell packing: A determinant of cell release. Blood. 46:91, 1975.
11. Lichtman, MA, Chamberlain, JK, Simon, W, Santillo, PA. The parasinosoidal location of megakaryocytes in marrow: A determinant of platelet release. Amer. J. Hemat. 4:303, 1978.
12. Lichtman, MA, Weed, RI. Alteration of the cell periphery during granulocyte maturation: Relationship to cell functions. Blood. 39:301, 1972.
13. Giordano, GF, Lichtman, MA. Marrow cell egress: The central interaction of barrier pore size and cell maturation. J. Clin. Invest. 52:1154, 1973.
14. Lichtman, MA. The ultrastructure of the hemopoietic environment of the marrow: A review. Exp. Hemat. 9:391-410, 1981.
15. DeBruyn, PPH, Michelson, S, Becker, RP. Endocytosis, transfer tubules and lysosomal activity in myeloid sinusoidal endothelium. J. Ultrastruct. Res. 53:133, 1975.
16. Chamberlain, JK and Lichtman, MA. Marrow cell egress: Specificity of the site of penetration into the sinus. Blood. 52:959, 1978.
17. DeBruyn, PPH and Michelson, S. An anionic material at the advancing front of blood cells entering the bone marrow circulation. Blood. 57:152, 1981.

MOVEMENT OF LEUKOCYTES IN FLOWING BLOOD

MARY P. WIEDEMAN

The fact that leukocytes adhere to the intraluminal
surface of blood vessels has long been noted as a point
of interest, yet the physiological significance of this
event remains undetermined. Although the microscopic
observations in vivo of these interesting cells to date
has been rewarding, leukocyte behavior in the living animal needs further study. There are three major aspects of
leukocyte behavior that can be investigated in this
manner; first, the adherence of leukocytes to the endothelial lining of vessels, second the motility of the cells
both inside and outside the vessels, and third, the hemodynamic forces which affect both the adherence and the
movement of the cells.

The information presented in this paper is a com-
pilation of the results of microscopic observations of the
microvessels in the bat wing and in the hamster cheek
pouch and deals primarily with factors which initiate or
inhibit leukocyte adherence.

Research leukocyte adherence in this laboratory was
initiated by Dr. Harvey Mayrovitz in 1975 with studies
designed to increase leukocyte adhesiveness by a discrete
thermal injury produced by a laser beam (1). The
following information was garnered from this study and
from subsequent investigations designed by Dr. Mayrovitz.

Leukocyte adherence is not normally seen in arterial
vessels of the bat wing or the hamster cheek pouch, but is
a common occurence in venous vessels and occasionally in

arterial vessels following surgical preparation of a tissue for microscopic observation.

Following mechanical occlusion of an arterial vessel, leukocytes will adhere to the vessel wall near the occlusion site but will not re-attach downstream once dislodged. This suggests that the adherence depends on alterations in the vessel wall and the leukocyte in the region of injury. (2)

While stasis of blood flow does not initiate adherence, it enhances pre-existing adherence. In arteriolar vessels with diameters of 15 to 40 um and red blood cell velocities of 1.1 to 4.4 $mmsec^{-1}$, if shear stress exceeds 8 $dynes/cm^2$, leukocytes will not adhere. (3)

Leukocytes adhered to arteriolar walls following laser injury in the adjacent interstitial space. The latent period between injury and adherence was inversely related to the surface area of injury and to the distance of the injury from the vessel wall. (4).

Adherence after injury in the interstitial space was thought to result from the diffusion of a chemotactic substance from the injury site to the vessel wall. The substance was not identified, but had a diffusion coefficient suggestive of a high molecular weight substance. There are numerous chemotactic materials liberated from injured tissue that could be responsible for causing leukocyte adherence.

In the course of a study of the action of sulfinpyrazone, a non-steroidal, anti-inflammatory drug, on platelet aggregation it was noted that in addition to reducing the duration of platelet activity at the site of an aggregate, sulfinpyrazone reduced the adhesiveness of leukocytes to vessel walls (5). The presence of these cells adhering or rolling along the wall, or accumulating in the immediate interstitial space are considered to indicate a response to injury or to signal an inflammatory response When it was noted that only a very few leukocytes were

visible in the vessels of animals that had been given
sulfinpyrazone prior to tests for the effects on platelet
behavior, it seemed possible that the drug could be
exerting a protective effect on the endothelial lining of
the blood vessels and therefore the adherence of leukocytes was diminished. Alternatively the drug could be
exerting an effect on the surface of the leukocyte.
Intravenous injections of sulfinpyrazone given after
surgical preparation of the pouch produced no significant
difference in the number of adhering leukocytes when compared to control animals. However, when intraperitoneal
injections 100 mgs/kg, were given each day for two days
and again one hour before preparation of the pouch, there
was a significant decrease compared to control values in
the number of leukocytes seen at the first reading and a
continued decrease through the first hour and a half so
that at 2 and $1/2$ hours, the leukocyte flux was less than $1/2$
the control value of the same time period. This appears
to be strong evidence that pretreatment with sulfinpyrazone modifies either the endothelial lining of the
vessels or the leukocytes themselves in such a way that
the factors responsible for adhesion are inhibited.

   Another aspect of sulfinpyrazone action is that it
alters the motility, and therefore the shape, of intravascular leukocytes. When a bolus of sulfinpyrazone was
injected into an arterial vessel to which leukocytes were
adhering, it was seen that the leukocytes became spherical
and rigid and could no longer maintain a "foothold" on the
vessel wall. Leukocytes that entered the observed area
seem unable to attach to the intraluminal surface of the
vessel, but bounced off the wall back into the blood
stream. Time-lapse photography revealed that the affected
leukocytes had no pseudopods that could extend and permit
the cell to adhere and crawl along the intraluminal surface of the vessel. This movement was frequently
retrograde to blood flow and must require considerable

energy for the cell to stick to the wall and move against
the vigorous arterial stream. It cannot be determined
from these experiments whether sulfinpyrazone is acting on
the vessel wall so that it loses its attractive force, or
whether it is acting on the leukocyte to render it unable
to respond to a chemotactic force. In any event, the drug
is effective in reducing leukocyte adherence to the intraluminal surface of arterial and venous vessels which have
been subjected to mild trauma.

The behavior of leukocytes as seen using in vivo
microscopy recorded on 16 mm color film using both regular
speed and time lapse, and many of the responses described
here can be seen in these movies.

References

1. Mayrovitz, H.N., Wiedeman, M.P., and Ascanio, G.:
    Changes in leukocyte adhesiveness accompanying laser
    irradiation. Fed. Proc. 34: 385, 1975.
2. Mayrovitz, H.N., Tuma, R.F. and Wiedeman, M.P.:
    Effect of stasis on leukocyte activity in micro-
    vessels. Biblio. Anat. 16: 403-405, 1977.
3   Mayrovitz, H.N. and Wiedeman, M.P.: Leukocyte adhesi-
    veness as influenced by blood velocity.
    Microcirculation 1: 128-129, 1976, Plenum Press.
4. Mayrovitz, H.N., Tuma, R.F. and Wiedeman, M.P.:
    Leukocyte Adherence in Arterioles following
    Extravascular Tissue Trauma. Microvas. Res. 20:
    264-274, 1980.
5. Wiedeman, M.P.: Microscopic Observation of Small
    Blood Vessels in Sulfinpyrazone-treated Animals. In:
    Cardiovascular Actions of Sulfinpyrazone: Basic and
    Clinical Research, Eds. McGregor, M., Mustard, J.F.,
    Oliver, M.F., and Sherry, S. Symposia Specialists,
    Inc. Miami, Florida, 99-112, 1980.

THE RELATIONSHIP BETWEEN LEUKOCYTE AND ERYTHROCYTE VELOCITY
IN ARTERIOLES

HARVEY N. MAYROVITZ

Introduction

Geometrical, rheological and functional differences between erythrocytes and leukocytes may give rise to differences in the in vivo flow dynamics of these two cellular
components of blood. One index which may shed light on
specific differences, if present, is the ratio of leukocyte
velocity (Vwbc) to erythrocyte velocity (Vrbc) in small
arterioles. No systematic study of the relationship
between these two quantities or the possible exploitation
of a demonstrated correlation between them has been
reported. Further, when such measurements are made simultaneously in vessels not significantly larger than leukocyte
dimensions the deviation of Vwbc/Vrbc from unity might provide a measure of an in vivo flow variance attributable to
some differential aspect between the two cellular
components. The purpose of the work reported here was to
investigate the relationship between Vrbc and Vwbc in small
arterioles and to establish base line data on the normally
occuring statistical distribution of the ratio of these two
quantities.

Methods

Eight female hamsters (110-140 gms) anesthetized with
pentabarbitol (.06mg/gm IP) were prepared for microscopic
observation of the cheekpouch vasculature which was exposed
and everted using standard techniques(1). An arteriole not
greater than 15um in diameter was selected for study and

Vrbc determined continuously for a period of 60 minutes using the photo-optic/crosscorrelation method(2,3). Simultaneously the microscopic image of the arteriole was recorded on video tape at an optical magnification of approximately 720 using a nuvicon TV camera and a BG/28 glass filter chosen to enhance the contrast of the leukocytes. Vwbc was determined by sensing the transit of each cell over a known axial distance using two cursors inserted into the video image of the arteriole. The electronic output of each cursor was displayed on a chart recorder and thereby permitted the determination of transit time and hence the calculation of Vwbc.

Each 60 minute experiment was divided into 240 consecutive intervals of 15 seconds duration. For each interval the number of leukocytes (wbc flux) and their velocity were determined. The average Vwbc in each interval was compared with the average Vrbc over the same interval by forming the ratio Vwbc/Vrbc. Statistical techniques were used to evaluate the distribution of this ratio within single and multiple intervals.

Results

One of the principle results of the present study is the demonstration of a very small difference between red blood cell velocity (Vrbc) and white blood cell velocity (Vwbc) simultaneously determined in arterioles with diameters ranging from 6.8 to 13.5 um. Based on 20,485 separate Vwbc measurements the average ratio Vwbc/Vrbc determined for all vessels was found to be 0.95± 0.06 (mean ± SD) as summarized in Table 1. This close agreement between Vwbc and Vrbc persisted despite an eight-fold variation in Vrbc and more than a three-fold variation in systemic wbc count.

TABLE 1. DATA SUMMARY - PARAMETERS AND RANGES

Diameter(um)	Vrbc(mm/sec)	WBC Count	# of WBCs	Vwbc/Vrbc
6.5-13.5	0.30-2.40	2600-7900	20,485	0.95±0.06

As an illustration of the relative constancy of the Vwbc/Vrbc ratio, Figure 1 summarizes the data obtained in one experiment from a 12.9 um diameter arteriole in which Vrbc varied from 0.4 to 1.8 mm/sec over the course of the measurement period (60 mins).

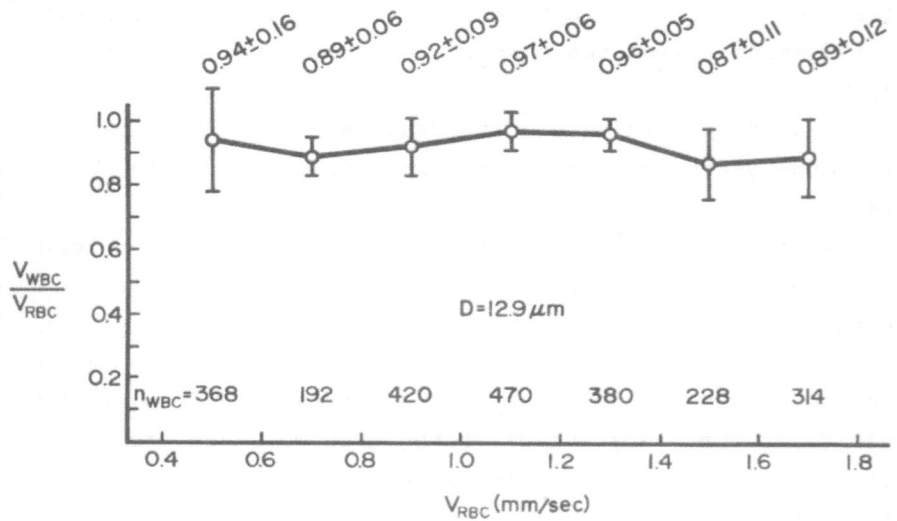

FIGURE 1. Ratio of Vwbc to Vrbc determined over the course of 60 minutes in an arteriole with large excursions in blood velocity. Data are for Vrbc ± 0.10mm/sec. Ratio = mean ± SD.

The velocity variations occurred spontaneously and without change in the diameter of the observed vessel. Utilizing this fortuitous spontaneous velocity change and by choosing contiguous Vrbc bins of 0.2 mm/sec width, one could determine the number of wbc's measured (n) within each quantized velocity range. For each group the average Vwbc/Vrbc ratio so calculated could then be expressed as shown in Figure 1. As may readily be seen, Vwbc/Vrbc was not less than 0.87, nor after calculation was there any statistical difference between velocity ratios as determined by analysis of variance. Further results demonstrating the close correspondence between Vrbc and Vwbc are shown in

Figure 2, which summarizes the data of four separate
experiments.

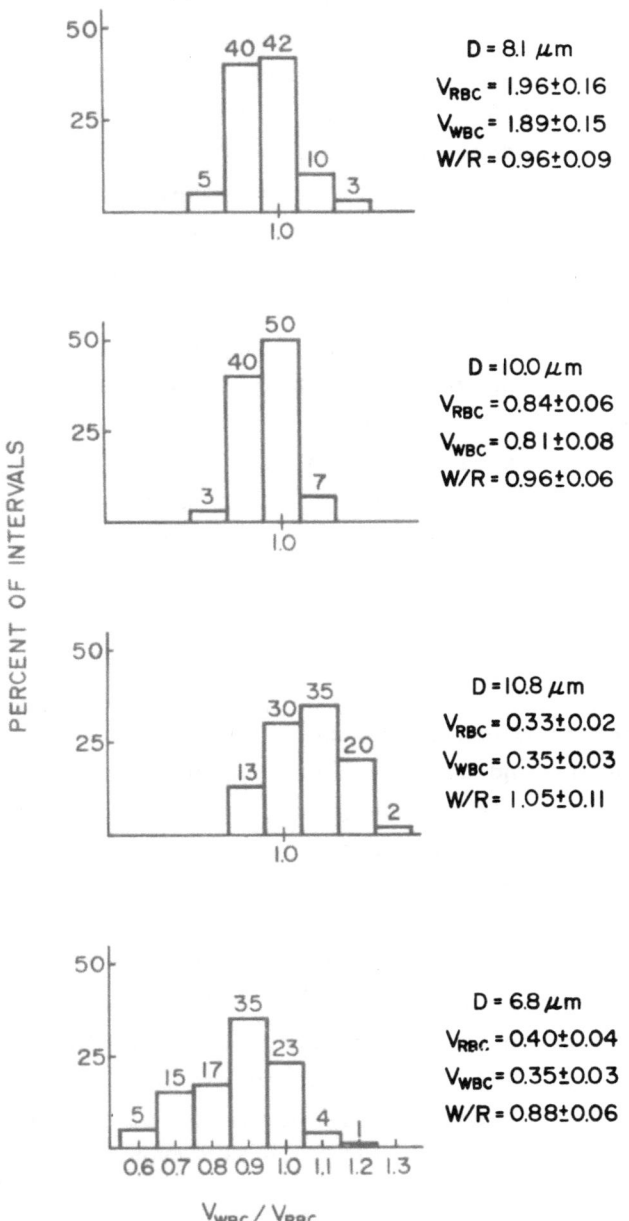

FIGURE 2.   Frequency distribution of Vwbc/Vrbc for widely
varying hemodynamic conditions.

The cases selected for presentation in Figure 2 were chosen so as to well illustrate the distribution of Vwbc/Vrbc for fairly wide hemodynamic and arteriole diameter differences.

Each histogram shows the percentage of the 240 separate 15-second intervals in which the Vwbc/Vrbc ratio was between the indicated ranges. The top panel, which illustrates a high Vrbc and intermediate diameter case, shows for example that in 82% of the intervals the Vwbc/Vrbc ratio was between 0.85 and 1.05. The middle two panels, which are for data obtained from similar diameter arterioles but significantly different blood velocities, are similarly tightly distributed but with mean values slightly below and above the unity ratio.

The bottom panel shows the distribution associated with a low blood velocity occurring in the smallest diameter arteriole studied. The Vwbc/Vrbc ratio in this case is more widely distributed than the previous cases and though skewed more toward lower values the mean ratio of 0.88 still represents a Vwbc/Vrbc ratio only slightly deviant from unity.

Discussion

Insight into capillary and post-capillary wbc intravascular processes and its relationship to microvascular hemodynamics continue to emerge(4-8). Information and understanding of wbc dynamics in arterioles is less well developed. In medium size arterioles the dependence of wbc-vessel wall interaction phenomena on blood velocity (9,10), transient blood stasis (11), focal tissue trauma (12), and microvascular hemodynamics (13) has been clarified but little data on events in arterioles less than about 15um is available (14,15). This problem has been addressed in the present work with the main parameter of interest being the ratio of white blood cell velocity (Vwbc) to red blood cell velocity (Vrbc).

The data obtained from over 20,000 measurements of white blood cell velocity in terminal arterioles has shown that on the average Vwbc is in fact slightly less than the

value of red blood cell velocity determined using now
standard cross-correlation techniques. The value for
Vwbc/Vrbc of 0.95±0.06 obtained as the average of all data
suggests that the hemodynamic impact of the white cell under
normal conditions is minimal in the arteriole vessel size
range studied. However it must not be inferred that this
cellular component of blood is without hemodynamic effects.
Firstly, the present method determines the Vwbc/Vrbc ratio
with the wbcs present in the vessel in which the measurement
is made. Even though no significant deviation in this ratio
from its mean value was found as a function of the wbc flux
vessel (5-50 cells/min) the possibility that Vrbc would be
higher in wbc free vessels (and the converse) cannot be
ruled out. Further, significant flow retarding processes
may well be found in smaller diameter vessels; at critical
pre-capillary branch points; under conditions of reduced
pressure gradient; or under conditions of enhanced wbc
vessel wall adherence.

When, as in the present case, Vwbc is determined in the
absence of these possible complicating factors it can be
utilized as an effective index of the absolute value of mean
red blood cell velocity with a calibration factor to account
for the small deviation found.

The use of wbc tracking for the subjective evaluation
of retinal blood flow via the blue field entoptic method
(16) has already been utilized. The present work represents
the first analytical approach known to the author to in fact
establish its validity provided that the retinal capillaries
are greater than a critical diameter. The results of the
present work also show that under conditions in which Vrbc
cannot be determined directly, Vwbc will yield adequate
values for the absolute value of blood velocity and together
with diameter measurements allow calculation of blood flow.
Of special interest in this regard is when fluorescent
microscopy is utilized to study in vivo wbc dynamics in the
microvasculature. The low light levels available do not
readily permit Vrbc to be determined using correlation

methods.   This previous limitation can now be overcome and
simultaneous information on wbc dynamics and hemodynamics
can be reliably obtained.

REFERENCES
1. Duling, BR   1973. The preparation and use of the
   hamster cheek pouch for studies of the microcirculation.
   Microvasc.Res. 5:423-429.
2. Intaglietta M, Tompkins WR and Richardson DR. 1970.
   Velocity measurements in the microvasculature of the cut
   omentum by on-line method. Microvasc.Res. 2:462-473.
3. Wiedeman MP, Tuma RF and Mayrovita HN. 1981.
   Introduction to microcirculation, Academic Press.
4. Atherton and Born, GVR. 1972. Quantitative
   investigations of the adhesiveness of circulating
   polymorphonuclear leukocytes to blood vessel walls. J.
   Physiol (London) 222:447-473.
5. Atherton A and Born GVR. 1973. Relationship between the
   velocity of rolling granulocytes and that of blood flow
   in venules. J. Physiol (London) 223:157-165.
6. Schmid-Schoenbein GW, Fung YC, Zweifach BW. 1975.
   Vascular endothelium - leukocyte interaction. Circ.Res.
   36:173.
7. Schmid-Schonbein GW, Usami S, Skalak R, Chien S. 1979.
   The interaction of leukocytes and erythrocytes in
   capillary and post-capillary vessels. Microvasc.Res.
   19:45-70.
8. Bagge U, Karlsson R. 1980. Maintenance of white blood
   cell margination at the passage through small venular
   junctions. Microvasc.Res. 20:92-95.
9. Mayrovitz HN, Wiedeman MP. 1976. Leukocyte adhesiveness
   as influenced by blood velocity. Microcirculation Ed.
   Grayson and Zingg. 128-130. Plenum Press. NY.
10. Mayrovitz HN, DeBovis M, Roy J. 1979. Leukocyte and
    erythrocyte velocity in arterial microvessels.
    Microvasc.Res. 17(2):572.
11. Mayrovitz HN, Tuma RF, Wiedeman MP. 1977. Effect of
    stasis on leukocyte activity in microvessels. Bibl.Anat.
    (No.16) 403-405.
12. Mayrovitz HN, Tuma RF, Wiedeman MP. 1980. Leukocyte
    adherence in arterioles following extravascular tissue
    trauma. Microvasc.Res. 20:264-274.
13. Mayrovitz HN, Wiedeman MP, Tuma RF. 1977. Factors
    influencing leukocyte adherence in microvessels.
    Thromb.Haemostas 38:823-830.
14. Schmin-Schonbein, Skalak R, Usami, Chien S. 1980. Cell
    distribution in capillary networks. Microvasc.Res.
    19:18-44.
15. Bagge U, Amundson B, Braide M. 1980. A method to observe
    and quantitate lekocyte interference with flow in the
    skeletal muscle microcirculation. Bibl.Anat.(No.20)
    557-560.
16. Sinclair SH, Loebl M, Riva CE. 1981. Blue field entoptic
    test in patients with ocular trauma. Arch.Ophth.
    99:464-467.

LEUKOCYTE PLUGGING OF CAPILLARIES *IN VIVO*

U.BAGGE and M.BRAIDE

The undeformed leukocyte is spherical.The average diameters
of lymphocytes,neutrophil granulocytes and monocytes are 6.2,
7.0 and 7.5 μm respectively (Schmid-Schönbein et al.,1980 a).
Although these diameters are considerably smaller than those
usually reported in hematology textbooks (10-20 μm),they are
still larger than those of most nutritive capillaries.For instance,in skeletal muscle the average capillary diameter is only
about 5 μm (Eriksson and Myrhage,1972).From these boundary conditions it follows that leukocytes must deform in order to be
able to circulate through the microvascular bed.

It is well-known that leukocytes are capable of both active
motion and spontaneous deformation.Observations of these phenomena show that the leukocytes undoubtedly can undergo very
large deformations;in inflammation the leukocytes may move through
gaps in the endothelium which are not wider than a few micra.
This active deformation is a comparatively slow process.Accor-
ding to e.g. Clark et al.(1936) the emigration of leukocytes
across the endothelium requires 2 to 9 minutes.Large deformations may take place in a much shorter time when the leukocytes
are passively deformed in the response to externally applied
stresses,such as the driving pressure in the circulation.Still,
the leukocytes do not by far adapt as quickly as the erythrocytes
to the varying dimensions of the microvasculature.Already under
normal flow conditions the leukocytes tend to interrupt or slow
down the blood flow in narrow capillaries.This effect of leukocytes on capillary perfusion is usually referred to as leukocyte

plugging (Fig.1).

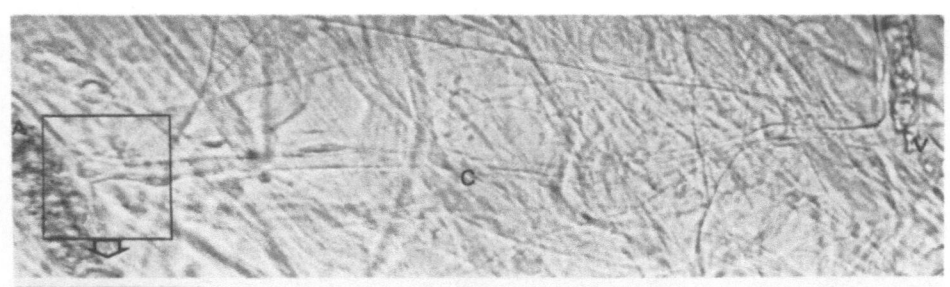

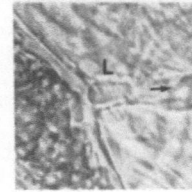

Figure 1.Leukocyte plugging (L) of a mesenteric capillary (C) in the rabbit.No other blood cells are present in the capillary.(A)-arteriole,(V)-venule.The arrow indicates the flow direction.

Krogh (1922) seems to have been the first to describe the different flow behaviour of leukocytes and erythrocytes in respect to their passage through the capillary bed.Thus,Krogh noticed that "the resistance offered to their (leukocytes) passage through vessels with diameters less than their own appeared to be greater than that experienced by the erythrocytes". A more comprehensive description of leukocyte behaviour in capillaries was published by Sandison (1932) on the basis of vital microscopic studies in the rabbit ear chamber.Sandison made the striking observation that even a single leukocyte was capable of completely stopping the circulation in a capillary.This blockage was usually located to the entrance of the small vessels. Although leukocytes were sometimes obstructing the flow for several minutes,Sandison concluded that the phenomenon was of minor importance since it was always temporary.

Nicoll and Webb (1946),who used the bat wing to visualize the microcirculation,were the first to recognize leukocyte plugging as an important cause of intermittent flow in capillaries. Further,these authors observed that leukocyte plugging was not mainly restricted to the entrance region of the vessels but that it occurred frequently also along the course of the vessels, preferrably where an endothelial cell nucleus protruded into

the lumen.Nicoll and Webb emphasize that "this type of plugging
by leukocytes occurs in normal fields with vigorous flow,and
is not related to leukocyte blockage that results from a developing tendency for them to adhere to the vascular walls".In
these authors opinion it is the dimensions,low pressure and al-
ternate routes of the capillary network that promotes leukocyte
plugging,whereas for instance Illig (1957) implies that leukocyte plugging is the result of sphincter action.Palmer (1959),
however,found no evidence of sphincter action in connection
with leukocyte plugging in the rat pancreas microcirculation
and remarks that "it is probable that some degree of leukocyte
plugging occurs whenever the diameter of the vessel is appreciably less than that of the leukocyte".Palmer points to the
risk of overlooking leukocyte plugging if a low optical magnification is used.This can lead to the misinterpretation that
intermittent flow in capillaries is caused by vascular contrac-
tions alone.Another two of Palmer´s observations should be mentioned,being of interest in some pathological situations to be
discussed later.Firstly,he noticed that the duration of leukocyte plugging was longer when the general flow was sluggish.
Secondly,that a sluggish flow increased the frequency of leukocyte plugging.To explain his latter finding,Palmer refers to
the *in vitro* experiments by Vejlens (1938).Vejlens´ studies indicate that the leukocytes (because of their size) flow nearer
the central stream of a tube when the flow is rapid,whereas at
low flow rates (where the erythrocytes tend to form aggregates)
the leukocytes would mainly flow in the marginal stream (see
also Palmer,1967.,Nobis,Pries,Gaehtgens,1981).Such a flow dependent radial distribution of the leukocytes would increase their
chances of entering,and blocking,capillary side branches in
low flow states.

When leukocytes block a capillary,the capillary does not seem
to collapse (Robb and Jabs,1968.,see also Figure 1).Although
it may seem that a plugging leukocyte is completely filling the
capillary lumen,not only plasma but also platelets and erythrocytes may sometimes manage to squeeze past the leukocyte
(Brånemark and Lindström,1963).Behind an obstructing leukocyte

erythrocytes often become packed together,whereas the plasma
flow past the leukocyte produces a cell-free plasma space at
its front.When the arrested leukocyte resumes its flow through
the vessel the erythrocytes follow closely behind,forming a
leukocyte-erythrocyte "train".The velocity of such a train or
of an individual leukocyte in a narrow capillary is usually much
slower than that of freely circulating erythrocytes (Asano et al.,
1973.,Schmid-Schönbein et al.,1980b.,Nobis and Gaehtgens,1980).

A detailed study of the rheology of human leukocytes *in vivo*
was performed by Bagge and Brånemark (1977)(see also Bagge,
1975).In these experiments high resolution vital microscopic
observations were made with a skin tube chamber technique (cf.
Brånemark,1971).Special attention was paid to the mode of deformation of the leukocytes and their shape changes in narrow
vessels.The studies show that leukocytes are deformed in a bi-
phasic manner.This behaviour was most clearly demonstrated when
the cells engaged a small (4-5 μm) capillary orifice.Then,in
a first step of very short duration (often less than 50 msec)
a tongue of the leukocyte would extend into the capillary.After
this very rapid,but only partial adaptation to the vessel lumen would follow a much slower deformation (typically 0.5-3
sec),during which the leukocytes attained a cylindrical shape.
The viscoelastic properties of the leukocytes indicated by these
in vivo observations were further analysed,quantitatively,*in*
vitro by Bagge et al.(1977b) and quite recently also by Schmid-
Schönbein et al.(1981).Both studies show that the viscoelastic
properties of the leukocytes can be represented by a standard
solid model,i.e. a spring in parallel with a Maxwell element,
containing another spring in series with a viscous element (Figure 2).

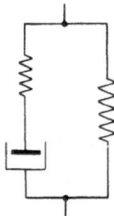

Figure 2.Standard solid viscoelastic model for leukocytes.

The degree of deformation which the leukocytes undergo when traversing a capillary is sometimes considerable.In one case Palmer (1959) observed a leukocyte which was transformed into a cylinder 40 μm long and 5 μm in diameter.Since the leukocytes deform in capillaries without any appreciable change in volume (Bagge and Brånemark,1977.,Bagge et al.,1977b) such extensive deformations of the originally spherical leukocyte imply large increases in surface area (as much as 60%).However,the leukocytes have much more membrane area than is needed to enclose their volume,in the form of fine membrane foldings Bagge et al., 1977a.,Schmid-Schönbein et al.,1980a).Consequently,the leukocytes can undergo large deformations without actual change in area;during passage through narrow capillaries the leukocytes simply unfold the membrane (Bagge et al.,1977a).

There is clearly enough experimental evidence to state that leukocytes must be taken into account when considering the factors influencing the distribution and velocity of blood flow in the microcirculation.However,leukocyte plugging is normally too rare a phenomenon and usually of too short duration to be harmful in respect to the nutrition of the tissues.It is easy to point at pathological conditions where the situation might be different.

In leukemia not only leukocyte numbers may be increased but also the cell rigidity.Lichtman and Weed (1972) applied a micropipette technique to study the deformability of normal leukocytes;Lichtman (1973) used the same technique to study the deformability of leukemic lymphoblasts and myeloblasts.Together, these experiments indicate that leukemic cells are much more rigid than normal leukocytes.Thus,while normal cells require only about 10 mm H_2O suction pressure to be partly drawn into a pipette with a 3.5 μm opening,a comparable deformation of e.g. leukemic myeloblasts into a 5 μm pipette requires as much as 250 mm H_2O negative pressure. Such pronounced rigidity of the leukemic cells certainly seems incompatible with normal transit of the cells through the microvasculature.As a result,leukemic cells may,particularly at high leukocrits,cause significant disturbances of capillary perfusion and tissue nutrition.

Lichtman (1973) even speculates that "several symptoms of leukemia whose pathogenesis is unexplained,such as joint,bone and
abdominal pain and episodes of tissue infarction may be a consequence of leukocclusive events".

As mentioned earlier,Palmer (1959) noticed that the frequency and duration of leukocyte plugging seemed to increase in
situations of sluggish flow in the microcirculation.These observations clearly suggest that a second mechanism promoting
leukocyte plugging is associated with low pressure gradients
in the capillary bed.

In hemorrhagic shock,where perfusion pressures may be substantially reduced (Mellander and Lewis,1963),leukocyte plugging
is mainly found in the pulmonary and skeletal muscle microvas-
culature.In the lungs of cat and dog,hemorrhage has been shown
to cause a large increase in the number of leukocytes trapped in
alveolar capillaries,and,in addition,in the number of leukocytes adhering to the endothelium in arterioles and venules (Wilson et al.,1970,Wilson,1972).Vital microscopic experiments in our laboratory show that hemorrhagic shock produces similar leukocyte phenomena in cat skeletal muscle (Eriksson and Lisander,
1972.,Ericson and Eriksson,1973.,Amundson et al.,1980.,Bagge
et al.,1980).On the basis of these studies we have concluded
that there is a causal connection between leukocyte plugging
and the heterogenous capillary perfusion which is observed in
skeletal muscle *in vivo* and which is also indicated in whole
organ studies by isotope clearance techniques in hemorrhagic
shock (Appelgren,1972.,Dahlberg,1979).

A major question is that of the quantitative importance of
leukocyte plugging in respect to the nutritive flow in shock.
Lipowsky et al.(1980) analysed the flow *in vivo* in individual
microvessels of the cat mesentery and found that leukocyte adhesion causes a large increase of the flow resistance in low
flow situations. Experiments in progress in our laboratory seem
to confirm a strong influence of leukocytes on the microvascular blood flow in situations with low driving pressures.

In order to quantitate the significance of leukocyte blockage in the skeletal muscle microcirculation we utilize the

isolated rat hindquarter preparation and isogravimetric technique (cf.Folkow et al.,1974).The hindquarter preparation,which
is perfused with a Tyrode-albumin-dextran solution (290 mOsmol/l),
allows calculation of capillary filtration coefficient (CFC)
and vascular resistance at different flow conditions. In our
experiments a bolus of homologous leukocytes ($5 \cdot 10^5$ to 10^6)
have been added to the cell free perfusate at flows ranging
from 0.9 to 8 ml/minx100g.In early experiments leukocytes were
separated from whole blood using a medium containing sodium
metrizoate and methylcellulose (see Bagge et al.,1977 b).With
this method infusion of leukocytes consistently gave at least
80-100% increase in vascular resistance and a decrease of the
CFC by as much as 60-70% in the low flow range (0.9-1.5 ml/minx100g)
(Bagge et al.,1981).A very small effect was found at the highest flow rates.However,these results must be taken with caution
since recent experiments,using a different method for leukocyte
separation (Ficoll 400 + sodium metrizoate),have shown only
about 20-30% increase in vascular resistance at the low flows.
The effects of leukocytes at the high flow rates were insigni-
ficant also in these experiments,which is consistent with the
concept that leukocyte plugging is a pressure dependent phe-
nomenon.It is obvious,however,that further experiments are required to establish the true level of effectiveness for leukocyte plugging in the skeletal muscle microcirculation.

REFERENCES

Amundson,B.,Jennische,E. and Haljamäe,H. Correlative analysis
    of microcirculatory and cellular metabolic events in skeletal
    muscle during hemorrhagic shock. Acta Physiol Scand 108,147-
    158,1980.
Appelgren,K.L.Capillary transport in relation to perfusion pres-
    sure and capillary flow in hyperemic dog skeletal muscle in
    shock. Eur.Surg.Res.8,311-320,1972.
Asano,M.,Brånemark,P-I. and Castenholz,A. A comparative study
    of continuous qualitative and quantitative analysis of micro-
    circulation in man. Microchymography and microphotoelectric
    plethysmography applied to microvascular investigation.

Adv.Microcirc. 5,1-31,1973.

Bagge,U. White Blood Cell Rheology.Experimental studies on
the rheological properties of white blood cells in man and
rabbit and in an *in vitro* micro-flow system. Dissertation,
University of Göteborg,1975.

Bagge,U. and Brånemark,P-I. White blood cell rheology.An intravital study in man. Adv.Microcirc. 7,1-17,1977.

Bagge,U.,Johansson,B.R. and Olofsson,J. Deformation of white
blood cells in capillaries. A combined intravital and electron microscopic study in the mesentery of rabbits. Adv.
Microcirc. 7,18-28,1977a.

Bagge,U.,Skalak,R. and Attefors,R. Granulocyte rheology.Expe-
rimental studies in an *in vitro* micro-flow system. Adv.
Microcirc. 7,29-48,1977b.

Bagge,U.,Amundsson,B. and Lauritzen,C. White blood cell deformability and plugging of skeletal muscle capillaries in hemorrhagic shock. Acta Physiol Scand 108,159-163,1980.

Bagge,U.,Amundson,B. and Braide,M. A method to observe and
quantitate leukocyte interference with flow in the skeletal
muscle microcirculation. 11th Europ.Conf.Microcirculation,
Garmisch-Partenkirchen 1980. Biblthca anat.,20,557-560
(Karger-Basel),1981.

Brånemark,P-I. Intravascular anatomy of blood cells in man
(Karger-Basel/New York),1971.

Brånemark,P-I. and Lindström,J. Shape of circulating blood
corpuscles. Biorheology,1,139-142,1963.

Clark,E.R.,Clark,E.L. and Rex,R.O.Observations on polymorphonuclear leukocytes in the living animal. Amer.J Anat.57,
385-438,1936.

Dahlberg,B. Blood-tissue solute exchange in skeletal muscle
during shock and trauma.Dissertation,University of Göteborg.
Acta Physiol Scand 1979,Suppl.472.

Eriksson,E. and Lisander,B. Low flow states in the microvessels
of skeletal muscle in cat. Acta Physiol Scand 86,202-210,1972.

Eriksson,E. and Myrhage,R. Microvascular dimensions and blood
flow in skeletal muscle. Acta Physiol Scand 86,211-222,1972.

Ericson,L.E. and Eriksson,E. Morphological aspects of intra-
and extravascular phenomena in cat skeletal muscle in cat.
Adv.Microcirc.5,72-79,1973.

Folkow,B,Hallbäck,M.,Lundgren,Y.,Weiss,L.,Albrecht,I. and
Julius,S. Analysis of design and reactivity of series -
coupled vascular sections in spontaneously hypertensive
rats (SHR). Acta Physiol Scand 90,654-656,1974.

Illig,L. Capillar "Contractilität",Capillar "Sphincter" und
"Zentralkanäle". Klin.Wschr. 35,7-22,1957.

Krogh,A. The Anatomy and Physiology of Capillaries. Hafner
Publ.Co.,New York (1922),Ed.of 1959.

Lichtman,M.A. Rheology of leukocytes,leukocyte suspensions and
blood in leukemia. J.Clin.Invest.52,350-358,1973.

Lichtman,M.A. and Weed,R.I. Alteration of the cell periphery
during granulocyte maturation:relationship to cell function.
Blood,39,301-316,1972.

Lipowsky,H.H.,Usami,S. and Chien,S. In vivo measurements of
"apparent viscosity" and microvessel hematocrit in the mesentery of the cat. Microvasc.Res.19,297-319,1980.

Mellander,S. and Lewis,D.H. Effect of hemorrhagic shock on the
reactivity of resistance and capacitance vessels and on capillary filtration transfer in cat skeletal muscle.Circulat.
Res.13,105-118,1963.

Nicoll,P.A. and Webb,R.L. Blood circulation in the subcutaneous
tissue of the living bat´s wing.Ann.N.Y.Acad.Sci.46,697-711,
1946.

Nobis,U. and Gaehtgens,P. Effect of white blood cells(WBC) on
blood rheology in narrow tubes. Abstract.Microvasc.Res.19,
395-396,1980.

Nobis, U., Pries, A. R. and Gaehtgens, P. Rheological mechanism
contributing to WBC-margination. 1981
this work-shop

Palmer,A.A. A study of blood flow in minute vessels of the pan-
cratic region of the rat with reference to intermittent cor-
puscular flow in individual capillaries.Quart.J.Exptl.Phys.
44,149-159,1959.

98

Palmer,A.A. Platelet and leukocyte skimming.Biblthca anat.,
    $\underline{9}$,300-303,$\underline{1967}$.(Karger,Basel/New York).
Robb,H.J. and Jabs,C. Distortion and dynamics of cellular ele-
    ments in the microcirculation. Angiology,$\underline{19}$,602-611,$\underline{1968}$.
Sandison,J.C. Contraction of blood vessels and observations
    on the circulation in the transparent chamber in the rabbits
    ear. Anat.Rec.$\underline{54}$,105-127,$\underline{1932}$.
Schmid-Schönbein,G.W.,Shih,Y.Y. and Chien,S. Morphometry of
    human leukocytes. Blood,$\underline{56}$,866-875,$\underline{1980a}$.
Schmid-Schönbein,G.W.,Usami,S.,Skalak,R. and Chien,S. The inter-
    action of leukocytes and erythrocytes in capillary and post-
    capillary vessels. Microvasc.Res.$\underline{19}$,45-70,$\underline{1980b}$.
Schmid-Schönbein,G.W.,Sung,K-L.P.,Tözeren,H.,Skalak,R. andChien,S.
    Passive mechanical properties of human leukocytes. Biophys.J.
    $\underline{1981}$,In press.
Vejlens,G. The distribution of leukocytes in the vascular sys-
    tem. Acta Path.Microbiol.Scand.,Suppl.$\underline{33}$,11-239,$\underline{1938}$.
Wilson,J.W.,Ratliff,N.B. and Hackel,D.B. The lung in hemorrhagic
    shock. I. In vivo observations of pulmonary microcirculation
    in cats. Amer J Path,$\underline{58}$,337-353,$\underline{1970}$.
Wilson,J.W. Leukocyte sequestration and morphologic augmenta-
    tion in the pulmonary network following hemorrhagic shock
    and related forms of stress. Adv.Microcirc.$\underline{4}$,197-232,$\underline{1972}$.

Acknowledgement:This work was supported by grants from the
Swedish Medical Research Council (B81-12X-00663-16A).

LEUKOCYTE MOTION IN THE MICROCIRCULATION (COMMENTARY)

S. CHIEN

MOVEMENT OF LEUKOCYTE IN FLOWING BLOOD

This paper by Dr. Wiedeman presents a summary of the results obtained in her laboratory on the microscopic observations of the microvessels in the bat wing and the hamster cheek pouch, dealing primarily with factors which initiate or inhibit leukocyte adherence. The presentation was highlighted by the showing of an excellent motion picture, which unfortunately cannot be fully represented in words. The main features shown in the movie are the following:

1. The irregular pattern of leukocyte adherence in arterial vessels during high flow.
2. The deformation of leukocytes in narrow microvessels.
3. The deformation of leukocytes in lymphatics.
4. The relative absence of leukocytes in capillaries.
5. The pavement of leukocytes in veins following local injury.
6. The difficulty of dislodging adhered leukocytes with saline.
7. The active retrograde motion of leukocytes.
8. The decrease in leukocyte adherence by sulfinpyrazone.
9. The shape change of leukocytes and loss of pseudopods following sulfinpyrazone.

One of the interesting findings is that sulfinpyrazone reduces the adherence of leukocytes to vascular endothelium. The experimental results do not allow one to conclude whether sulfinpyrazone acts on the vessel wall or the leukocyte. It may be helpful to treat leukocytes with sulfinpyrazone _in vitro_ and then administer them to the microcirculation _in vito_. Alternatively, one can use the microperfusion technique to administer sulfinpyrazone to an occluded segment of venule in the absence of leukocytes and later study leukocyte adherence to the segment after flushing out the surfinpyravone.

THE RELATIONSHIP BETWEEN LEUKOCYTE AND ERYTHROCYTE VELOCITY IN ARTERIOLES

This paper presents quantative data on the relationship between red blood cell velocity (Vrbc) and white blood cell velocity (Vwbc) in 6.8 - 13.5 μm arterioles in the hamster cheek pouch. The results on the 20,485 Vwbc measurements yield a Vwabc/Vrbc ratio of 0.95 ± 0.06 (mean ± SD) over a range of Vrbc from 0.30 to 2.40 mm/sec. Grouping of data according to Vrbc (0.4 to 1.8 mm/sec) showed that the Vwbc/Vrbc ratio did not vary significantly with Vrbc and was not less than 0.87 in all groups.

Although the numerical value of the Vwbc/Vrbc ratio is closed to 1.0, the consistency of the finding that this ratio is less than 1 in all Vrbc groups (Figure 1) suggests that the difference is real. The significance of the difference of each Vwbc/Vrbc ratio from 1.0 can be evaluated with Student's t test, where the t value can be calculated as:

$$t = \frac{1 - M}{S.D. / \sqrt{N}}$$

For the various groups shown in Figure 1 the t value ranges from 7.19 (for the group with Vrbc = 0.5 mm/sec) to 254.0 (for the group with Vrbc = 0.7 mm/sec). These results indicate that the P value is less than 0.001 in all cases. That is, the Vwbc/Vrbc ratio is significantly lower than 1.0, or Vwbc is less than Vrbc, although by only 5 percent on the average. These results are in agreement with previous studies on the influence of leukocytes on the flow behavior of red blood cells in narrow vessels and narrow tubes. In narrow vessels with a diameter not markedly larger than the white cell diameter, the presence of a leukocyte often causes the formation of a train of red blood cells with close spacing behind the leukocyte, thus leading to close similarity in the velocity of these two types of cells (1). Nobis and Gaehtgens (2) have performed quantitative studies in vitro on the relationship between tube diameter and the probability of passage of red blood cells around the white blood cell. In a glass tube with 8 μm diameter no red blood cells can overtake the leukocyte. In tubes with larger diameters some of the red blood cells can pass the white blood cells; in a glass tube with 15 μm diameter only 3 percent of red blood cells are able to pass the white blood cells, and these single red blood cells have a velocity approximately 30 percent higher than that in the train behind the white blood cell. These results indicate that, in the range of vessel diameter studied in this paper, Vrbc and Vwbc should be close to each other, with the Vrbc being a little faster. Considering the difficulties involved in making the in vivo measurements, the results in this study agree remarkably well with those obtained in vitro. It is to be emphasized that the large number of measurements performed by the author made it possible to ascertain the significance of the small difference statistically.

The ability of the red blood cells to pass a white blood cell in a narrow vessel would depend on the degree of cell deformation in response to shear stress. Therefore, one might expect a dependence of Vwbc/Vrbc ratio on Vrbc. It is to be noted, however, that the ratio U of Vrbc to tube diameter ranges from 39 to 132 sec^{-1} for the data presented in Figure 1; these U values correspond to wall shear stress of 9 to 32 $dynes/cm^2$, respectively, which are probably sufficient to cause maximum red cell deformation.

In the Discussion section the author correctly pointed out that these data do not exclude the possibility that Vrbc would be higher in wbc-free vessels. If the presence of a wbc causes a significant decrease in Vrbc in comparison to that found in the absence of wbc, then the statement "the hemodynamic impact of the white cell under normal conditions is minimal in the arterial vessel size range studied" would have to be modified. By the same token, the conclusion that "Vwbc .... can be utilized as an effective index of the absolute value of mean red blood cell velocity" can be applied only to those situations where white cells are present in the narrow vessels studied.

In summary, this paper represents an important contribution to the understanding of the interrelationship between white blood cells and red blood cells in the microcirculation and it points out the need for further studies in this rapidly developing new area of investigation.

REFERENCES

1. Schmid - Schoenbein, G.W., Usami, S., Skalak, R. and Chien, S. The interaction of leukocytes and erythrocytes om capillary and post-capillary vessels. Microsvac. Res. 19: 45-70, 1980.
2. Nobis, U. and Gaehtgens, P. Rheology of white blood cells during blood flow through narrow tubes. Bibliotheca Anat. 20: 211-214, 1981.

LEUKOCYTE PLUGGING OF CAPILLARIES IN VIVO

This is an excellent concise review of the state of the art of our knowledge on the role of the mechanical properties of leukocytes in affecting microcirculatory flow in vivo. It places in perspective the physiological and pathophysiological significance of the in vitro tests on the viscoelastic properties of leukocytes presented in the earlier part of this workshop. The authors pointed out that, while leukocyte plugging is a rare phenomena under normal conditions, it may be of considerable significance in disease states such as leukemia and circulatory shock.

At the end of the paper, the authors give a brief description of the results of their experiments on the effect of leukocyte infusion on the flow resistance and capillary filtration coefficient in the isolated rat hindquarter preparation, using an isovolumetric technique. Although the written description is rather brief, this was covered much more extensively at the presentation. These experiments demonstrate directly the influence of leukocytes on the flow dynamics and transcapillary fluid shifts under well controlled experimental conditions. Particularly interesting is the finding that the effects of leukocytes are flow-dependent, being much more pronounced in low flow states. The larger influence of the leukocytes obtained by using sodium metrizoate and methylcellulose than those obtained by using Ficoll and sodium metrizoate suggests that abnormalities in leukocytes can be detected by using this preparation.

IN VITRO MEASUREMENT OF LEUKOCYTE ADHESIVENESS

GUNNAR HOPEN

Before leaving the circulation, the leukocytes must adhere to the vessel wall with a force sufficiently high to resist the shearing force of the flowing blood. This process depends on the presence of divalent cations, as demonstrated in vivo (1). To elucidate the role of the leukocyte in this process, various in vitro assays of leukocyte adhesiveness have been developed. However, conflicting results obtained with these techniques indicate that they are reflecting different phenomena.

Active cell adhesion is a dynamic process where the strenght of attachment increases during a period of time after the initial adhesion (2). This indicates that assays for leukocyte adhesiveness, utilizing cell adhesion to a substrate in the presence of the shearing force of a constant flow (3,4,5), have relevance only to the very early fase of adhesion. In other assays, however, the leukocytes are allowed to attach to the substratum in absence of flow before a force is applied to remove non-adherent and more or less loosly attached cells (6,7,8). Conceivably, these techniques involve the more advanced stages of the adhesion process, depending on the time lag before the detaching force is applied, and the strength of this force.

Most assays use non-biological substrata e.g. glass (3,4,6), plastic (9) and nylon (5,10). Some cell types adhere avidly to artificial surfaces by passive adsorption. However, proteins in the suspending medium will coat the substratum almost instantly (11) and modify cell adhesion (12). One aim of the present study was to examine how proteins modify active and passive adhesion in two assays of leukocyte adhesiveness utilizing adhesion in the presence of flow: i) a glass bead column assay (13), and ii) the nylon wool column assay described by MacGregor et al (5).

The results of leukocyte adhesiveness measurements might also be influenced by the presence of other formed blood elements in the test system.

We have shown that platelets influence the results of whole blood measurements of leukocyte adhesiveness in glass bead columns, but not when erythrocyte-free suspensions of leukocytes in plasma are used (14).

Another aim of the present study was to test a possible influence of platelets on the results of nylon wool column measurements of leukocyte adhesiveness.

MATERIAL AND METHODS

Blood.

Heparinized blood (18 i.u. per ml) was donated by healthy, non-fasting members of the hospital staff, of which non had taken any drugs for at least 10 days prior to sampling.

Leukocytes were isolated by dextran (60 mg/ml, Pharmacia, Sweden) sedimentation, and contaminating red cells were lysed with 0.15 M ammonium chloride for 10 min. After washing twice in a solution of 0.15 M sodium chloride and 2.5 U/ml heparin, the leukocytes (60 - 70% neutrophil granulocytes) were suspended to a concentration of $7 \times 10^9/l$ in autologous plasma or Hanks balanced salt solution (HBSS) with or without addition of bovine serum albumin (BSA) (Armour Pharmaceutical Company LTD, England), gelatine (Difco Laboratories, Detroit, Michigan, U.S.A.) or autologous plasma.

Plasma was obtained by centrifugating heparinized blood for 10 min at 175 x g (platelet-rich) or for 30 min at 3500 x g (platelet-poor).

Platelet-poor blood was obtained by centrifugating whole blood for 10 min at 175 x g. The platelet-rich supernatant was spirated and centrifuged for 30 min at 3500 x g to obtaine platelet-poor plasma which was remixed with the sediment of the first centrifugation. To obtain control blood with high platelet concentration, the platelet-rich supernatant was remixed with its own sediment.

Measurement of leukocyte adhesiveness.

The nylon wool column assays was performed according to MacGregor et al (5). Pasteur pipettes were packed with a specified weight of scrubbed nylon fiber (Fenwal Laboratories, Illinois, U.S.A.) to a height of 15 mm above the constriction of the pipette. Samples of one ml blood or leukocyte suspension were applied to the top of the columns and allowed to flow by gravity. By counting the pre- and postcolumn concentration of leukocytes, the percentage of leukocytes retained in the column could be calculated.

The glass bead column assay has been described in detail previously

(13,14). Polyvinyl columns (internal diameter: 5mm) were packed with 2.5 g glass beads (average diameter: 0.5 mm). Leukocyte suspensions were perfused through the columns at a constant flow rate until eluates of 0.5 ml were obtained. The retention of leukocytes was expressed in per cent of the precolumn concentration.

Both assays were performed at a constant temperatur of 37°C. The glass bead column assay was also performed at 5°C. Differential counting being the main source of method variance (15), was omitted when experiments with suspensions of identical leukocyte composition were compaired. Preparation of samples with high and low platelet concentration resulted in slight differences in leukocyte composition. Consequently, granulocyte retention was calculated in these experiments. Differential counts were performed in May-Grünwald-Giemsa stained blood films or cyto-centrifuge preparations of leukocyte suspensions. To avoid cell aggregation, a final concentration of 10 mM sodium EDTA was added to precolumn samples for counting, and to postcolumn collection vials.

Statistical methods. Wilcoxon's paired sample test and Wilcoxon's one sample test were used for statistical analysis.

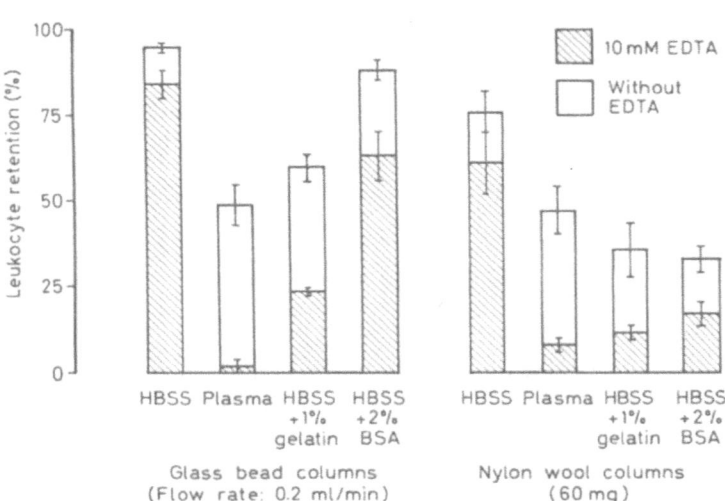

FIGURE 1. Leukocyte retention in glass bead- and nylon wool columns. Effect of the presence of proteins and EDTA in the suspending medium. Mean $\pm$ SEM, n:6.

RESULTS

In both glass bead- and nylon wool columns, a high retention of
leukocytes occurred after the passage of protein free leukocyte suspensions,
and chelation of divalent cations by adding EDTA to the suspensions
reduced leukocyte retention only slightly (Fig. 1). Addition of proteins
to the suspending medium decreased leukocyte retention and potentiated
the retention-inhibiting effect of EDTA. In suspensions of leukocytes
in autologous plasma, EDTA abolished the retention of leukocytes in
glass bead columns, whereas leukocyte retention in nylon wool columns
was significantly but not totally inhibited. Inhibition of leukocyte
retention by 2% BSA was stronger in nylon wool columns than in glass
bead columns. However, neither 2% BSA nor 1% gelatin did by far abolish
divalent-cation-independent retention of leukocytes in either columns
type. Aproximately the same results were obtained when serum was used
instead of plasma (data not shown).

Plasma inhibited leukocyte retention and potentiated the retention-
-inhibiting effect of EDTA in a dose response manner in both glass
bead- and nylon wool columns (Fig. 2).

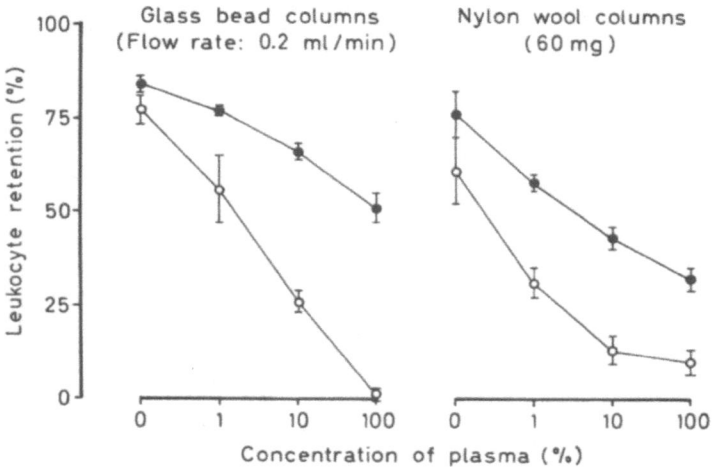

FIGURE 2. Leukocyte retention in glass bead- and nylon wool columns.
Effects of increasing concentrations of autologous plasma in suspensions
with 10 mM EDTA (o) and without (●). Mean $\pm$ SEM, n:6.

By decreasing the flow rate through glass bead columns, or increasing
the weigth of fiber in the nylon wool columns, the retention of leukocytes
from leukocyte-plasma suspensions increased in both column types (Fig. 3).

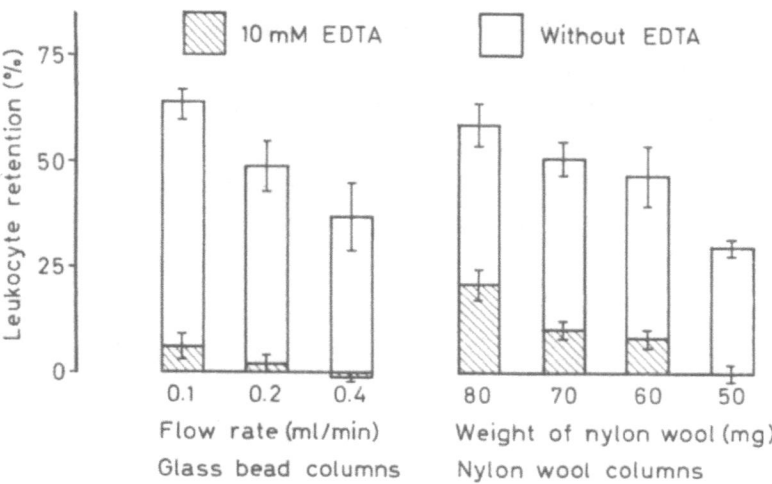

FIGURE 3. Leukocyte retention in glass bead- and nylon wool columns.
Effect of flow rate (glass bead columns) and weight of nylon wool (nylon
wool columns). Suspending medium: autologous plasma with or without
EDTA. Mean $\pm$ SEM, n:6.

In the glass bead columns, increased leukocyte retention was mainly
due to divalent-cation-dependent adhesion since no significant retention
was observed from EDTA-treated suspensions (P$>$0.1). However, a significant
retention of leukocytes from EDTA-treated suspensions occurred in 70
and 80 mg nylon wool columns (P=0.05), and no increase in divalent-
-cation-dependent adhesion was observed when the weight of nylon fiber
was increased beyond 60 mg.

Table 1. Effect of temperature on the retention in glass bead columns
of leukocytes suspended in plasma or HBSS (mean $\pm$ SEM).

Suspending medium	37°C	5°C	P-value
HBSS (n: 7)	93 $\pm$ 1	92 $\pm$ 1	$>$0.1
Plasma (n: 7)	45 $\pm$ 6	20 $\pm$ 2	=0.02

Leukocyte retention in glass bead columns was temperature-dependent
when the leukocytes were suspended in plasma, but not when suspended in
HBSS (Table 1).

Retention of granulocytes in nylon wool columns was significantly
higher after the passage of whole blood with high platelet concentration
compaired to blood with reduced platelet concentration. However,
granulocyte retention from suspensions of leukocytes in plasma was not
influenced by the concentration of platelets (Fig. 4).

Platelet retenion from platelet-rich whole blood (n: 6) was
(mean $\pm$ SEM): 85 $\pm$ 3, and from suspensions of leukocytes in platelet-rich
plasma: 20 $\pm$ 6 (n: 9).

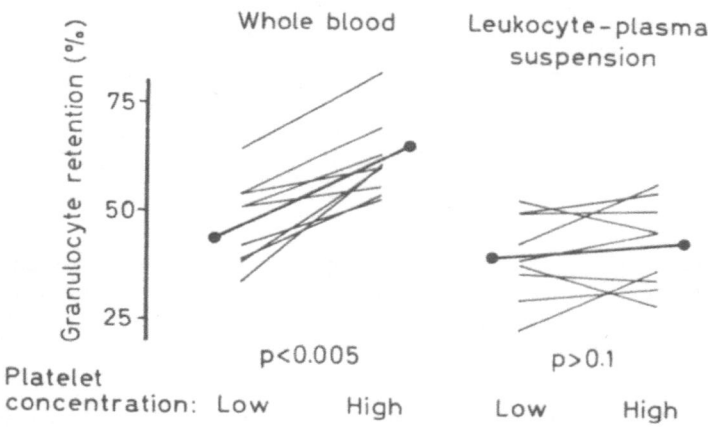

FIGURE 4. Granulocyte retention in nylon wool columns (70 mg).
Effect of platelet concentration (mean $\pm$ SEM x 10^9/l) in whole blood
(low: 87 $\pm$ 17 and high: 210 $\pm$ 15) and in suspensions of leukocytes in
autologous plasma (low: 23 $\pm$ 8 and high: 397 $\pm$ 49). N: 9.

DISCUSSION

Both assays of leukocyte adhesiveness studied involv the early fase of
leukocyte adhesion by measuring the retention of leukocytes after the
passage of heparinized whole blood or leukocyte suspensions through columns
packed with nylon wool (5) or glass beads (13). Previous studies on the
glass bead column assay revealed that highly different phenomena influenced
the retention of the leukocytes depending on experimental conditions like
the presence of other formed blood elements or proteins in the test system

(13,14,15,16). The possibility of a similar influence of these conditions on the results obtained with the nylon wool column assay was tested in the present study.

Cell adhesion to non-biological substrata depends mainly on the physico-chemical properties of the substratum like wettabily and surface charge (17,18). However, these properties are drastically changed when proteins from the cell suspending medium are adsorbed to the substratum (11). Taylor (12) showed that human conjunctiva cells, wether living or killed, attached rapidly to clean glass by a passive process, whereas cell adhesion to protein coated glass is a dynamic process depending on activity of the living cell. Taylor (12) and others, using different cell types (2,19,20) have demonstrated that active- but not passive adhesion is dependent on divalent cations. It therefor seems warranted to use dependence or independence of divalent cations as a criterion for active or passive adhesion respectively. When this criterion is applied on results obtained in previous studies, one may conclude that rat leukocytes (21) as well as human leukocytes (16) adhere to glass beads passively in the absence of protein, but actively when plasma proteins are added to the suspending medium. This conclusion is supported by the finding in the present study that leukocyte retention in glass bead columns was temperature-dependent when the leukocytes were suspended in plasma, but not when the leukocytes were suspended in a protein-free medium (Table 1).

In the present study we demonstrated that adhesion to nylon wool- as well as glass bead columns was mainly passive in the absence of proteins (Fig. 1). The finding that passive adhesion was inhibitet to a different degree by various proteins is in accordance with the results of previous studies on other cell types (12,19). The considerable difference in adhesion-inhibition by albumin in glass bead- and nylon wool columns may be related to different adsorption of albumin to glass and nylon as a result of the physico-chemical properties of the two materials (22). However, it should be noticed that addition of 1% gelatin or 2% BSA (commonly used as the only protein substance in leukocyte suspensions) did not abolish passive leukocyte adhesion to either type of columns.

Conflicting results in previous studies concerning the influence of plasma (serum) on leukocyte adhesion (6,23,24) may be due to the fact that no discrimination was made between active and passive adhesion. In the present study plasma effectively inhibited passive adhesion whereas

active adhesion was higher in plasma-containing suspension than in any
other suspension examined. This indicates that plasma enhance active
adhesion in both column types.

Retention of leukocytes can be increased by decreasing the flow rate in
glass bead columns (4), or by increasing the weight of nylon fibers per column
in nylon wool columns (5). In the glass bead columns, the increased leukocyte
retention following the reduction of the flow rate was appearently due to
increased active adhesion since no significant passive retention occurred
at any flow rate (Fig. 3). However, a significant passive retention was
observed in 70 and 80 mg nylon columns, whereas increasing the weight of
nylon fiber beyond 60 mg did not increase active adhesion. The reason
for this phenomenon is not clear. Since the different amounts of nylon
wool occupy equal volumes in the columns, the columns containing greater
amounts of nylon wool must necessarily be tighter packed. The possibility
of passive trapping of leukocytes is therefor greater in these columns than
in the looser packed columns containing less amounts of nylon wool. Since
the glass bead columns are porous to spheres up to a diameter of 0.3 times
the diameter of the glass beads (25), retention by simple trapping is less
probable in the glass bead columns used in this study.

Rasp et al (26) and Hopen (15), independently showed that the retention
of granulocytes from whole blood in nylon wool columns depended on the
concentration of platelets in the blood. In the present study was
demonstrated that the retention of granulocytes from erythrocyte-free
suspensions of leukocytes in plasma was not influenced by the platelet
concentration (Fig. 4). This is in accordance with our previous
observation that platelets enhance the retention of granulocytes in glass
bead columns only when erythrocytes are present in the test system (14).
This may be due to the fact that erythrocytes highly increase the retention
of platelets in glass bead columns (27), and in nylon wool columns as
shown in the present study.

In conflict with our results, Rasp and coworkers (26) reported that
platelets enhance granulocyte retention in nylon wool columns, even in
the absence of erythrocytes. However, this phenomenon, wich was pronounced
in protein free suspensions, was less obvious when suspensions containing
50% plasma were used. This indicates that the enhancement of granulocyte
retention by platelets in absence of erythrocytes is related to passive
cell adhesion (vide supra).

The results obtained in the present study invite to the following suggestions concerning the nylon wool- and the glass bead column assays of leukocyte adhesiveness:

1. The phenomenon which one usually intends to measure, the early fase of active leukocyte-to-surface adhesion, is reflected by the retention of leukocytes in the glass bead columns or columns packed with 60 mg or less nylon wool after the passage of suspensions of leukocytes in plasma (or serum) through the columns.

2. Retention of leukocytes in columns packed with 70 mg nylon wool or more is partly due to a passive process, possibly trapping of leukocytes by the tightly packed nylon fibers.

3. Retention of leukocytes in glass bead- or nylon wool columns after the passage of leukocytes suspended in protein-free media is mainly due to passive adhesion. This passive process is only partly inhibited by the addition of 2% BSA, 1% gelatin or 10% plasma to the suspension.

4. Retention of leukocytes in glass bead- or nylon wool columns after the passage of heparinized whole blood through the columns is due to an interaction between erythrocytes, platelets and leukocytes.

REFERENCES

1. Atherton A & Born GVR, J. Physiol. 222; 447-474, 1972.
2. Grinnell F, Int. Rev. Cytol. 53; 65-144, 1978.
3. Garvin JE, J. Exp. Med. 114; 51-73, 1961.
4. Kvarstein B, Scand. J. Clin. Lab. Invest. 23; 259-270, 1969.
5. MacGregor RR, Spagnuolo PJ & Lentnek AL, N. Eng. J. Med. 291; 642-646,1974.
6. Bryant RE & Sutcliffe MC, Proc. Soc. Exp. Biol. Med. 141; 196-202, 1972.
7. Lichtman MA & Weed RI, Blood 39; 301-316, 1972.
8. Fehr J, in Greenwalt TJ & Jamieson GA (eds.) The granulocyte: function and clinical utilization. P. 243-258, 1977 Alan R. Liss, Inc., New York.
9. Gallin JI, Wright DG & Schiffmann E, J. Clin. Invest. 62; 1364-1374, 1978.
10. Spitler LE, Spath P, Cooper N & Fundenberg HH, Br. J. Haematol 29; 279-292, 1975.
11. Bruck SD, J. Biomed. Mater. Res. 8; 1-21, 1977.
12. Taylor AC, Exp. Cell. Res. (Suppl.) 8; 154-173, 1961.
13. Hopen G & Schreiner A, Scand. J. Haematol. 22; 219-225, 1979.
14. Hopen G, Scand. J. Haematol. 22; 226-234, 1979.
15. Hopen G, Scand. J. Haematol. (in press) 1981.
16. Schreiner A & Hopen G, Acta Path. Microbiol. Scand. Sect. C, 87; 333-340, 1979.

112

17. Baier RE, Shafrin EG & Zisman, Science 162; 1360-1368, 1968.
18. Maroudas NG, J. Theor. Biol. 49; 417-424, 1975.
19. Nordling S, Acta Path. Microbiol. Scand. Suppl. 192; 1967.
20. Tacheichi M, Exp. Cell Res. 68; 88-96, 1971.
21. Garvin JE, J. Cell Physiol. 72; 197-212, 1969.
22. Vromann L, Adams AL, Klings M, Fischer GC, Munoz PL & Solensky RP, N.Y. Acad. Sci. 283; 65-76, 1977.
23. Kvarstein B, Scand. J. Clin. Lab. Invest. 24; 4-48, 1969.
24. Penny R, Galton DAG, Scott JT & Eisen V, Brit. J. Haemat. 12; 623-632, 1966.
25. Blumenson LE, J. Cell. Physiol 70; 7-22, 1967.
26. Rasp FL, Clawson CC & Repine JE, J. Lab. Clin. Med. 97; 812-819, 1981.
27. Hellem AJ, Scand. J. Clin. Lab. Invest., Suppl. 51: 1960.

ADHESION OF GRANULOCYTES TO HUMAN CULTURED ENDOTHELIAL CELLS

A. COURILLON, M.P. WAUTIER, J.P. ABITA, J.L. WAUTIER.

ABSTRACT

Adhesion is an essential function of the leucocyte in physiological and pathological processes such as bacterial defence, inflammation and possibly thrombosis. We have studied
the adhesion (to plastic and to endothelial cells) of normal
human granulocytes and granulocyte precursors (promyelocytic
leukemia HL 60 cells) at various stages of differentiation.
Purified leukocytes were labelled with ^{51}Chromium, and added
to confluent human cultured endothelial cells obtained from
umbilical veins. The Petri dishes (35 mm) were washed 5 times
and the radioactivity measured in each wash. The remaining
leukocytes were removed by sodium hydroxide. The effect of
increasing concentrations of leukocytes was to linearly increase the adhesion to plastic but did not markedly increase
the adhesion to endothelial cells.
The adhesion of granulocyte precursors (promyelocytic leukemia HL 60 cells) was significantly lower than that of mature
granulocytes. The adhesion increased in parallel with the
differentiation of the cells into granulocytes. They adhered
more to endothelial cells than normal leukocytes but as normal to plastic.

1. INTRODUCTION

The interaction between granulocytes and vascular endothelial cells is one of the primary events in the inflammatory
response. The development of the technique for endothelial
cell culture has permitted an in vitro model of this phenomenon. We have used a radiometric technique and cultured endothelial cells derived from human umbilical veins to investigate the development of the adhesive properties of mature

myeloid cells obtained in vitro at different stages of differentiation.

2. MATERIALS AND METHODS

- Granulocyte Isolation :

Heparinized blood was obtained from normal healthy donors.
Granulocytes were isolated by Ficoll Hypaque sedimentation
and contaminating red cells removed by Dextran sedimentation
and hypotonic lysis (1). Isolated granulocytes were suspended in 0.15 M Nacl and labelled with ^{51}Cr (1μ Ci / 10^6 leukocytes) using the method of Gallin et al (1). Labelled leukocytes (98 % $\pm$ 2 granulocytes) were resuspended in Hank's
balanced salt solution (HBSS) containing 1,3 mM calcium and
0,4 mM Magnesium (Institut Pasteur Paris) with 5 g / l of
human albumin (centre national de transfusion Paris). Platelet concentrations in granulocytes preparation were less
than one platelet for one leucocyte.

- Preparation of endothelial cells

Endothelial cells were cultured according to the method
of Jaffe et al (2).
The cells from each human umbilical vein were seeded in
35 mm plastic dishes (lux Scientific Newbury Calif.) in a
concentration of 40 000 per square centimeter. The culture
medium was M 199 (Gibco Glasgow) with 20 % fetal calf serum
(Gibco). The medium was changed every two days until the
cells reached confluence in seven to nine days. The endothelial cell cultures were assessed for purity initially by
transmission microscopy and immunofluorescence with a specific antibody to human factor VIII related antigen and rou-
tinely by phase-contrast microscopy.

- Leukocytes adhesion

Endothelial cell cultures were washed once in HBSS with
albumin and labelled leukocytes (0,7 ml) were layered on duplicate plates.
After incubation at 37° for 30 minutes in a 5 % CO_2 atmosphere, non adhesive cells were removed by gentle aspiration
and endothelial cells were washed four times with 1 ml of

HBSS with albumin. The endothelial cells and the leukocytes attached to the endothelial cells were then lysed with the addition of 1 ml of NaOH 1 M. The radioactivity of each wash was measured in an autologic gamma counter (Abbott).

The adhesion was also tested on 35 mm empty plastic Petri dishes (Lux Scientific, Newbury Calif.) under the same conditions.

The total radioactivity initialy added for the assay was measured from the radioactivity of 0,7 ml of the ^{51}Cr labelled granulocytes suspension. In all experiments, the total radioactivity was also calculated from the sum of the radioactivity of the five washes. When the measured total was different from the calculated total, the calculated total was used for estimation of adhesion.

The results were expressed as the percentage of total radioactivity that remained after each wash :

$$\frac{T - (R_1 + R_2 + R_x)}{T} \times 100$$

Where R is the radioactivity in the wash (cpm), x the number of the wash and T the total radioactivity (cpm).

The results were also expressed as the number of adhering cells that remained after each wash : Number of cells initialy layered x % radioactivity (cpm) remaining after the wash.

- HL 60 cells

HL 60 cell line has been maintained in continuous suspension for 4 years and cells were (kindly provided by Dr GALLO Bethesda - U S A) in RPMI 1640 medium (Gibco Glasgow) supplemented with 20 % fetal calf serum (Gibco) and were incubated at 37° in a humified atmosphere with 5 % CO_2. Retinoic acid (Sigma) was dissolved in 95 % ethanol (vol/vol) and final concentration in culture medium was 10^{-6}M.

3. RESULTS

3.1. Adhesion of normal granulocytes to endothelial cells and to plastic.

After the fifth wash the mean adhesion was $1.76 \pm 0.2 \times 10^6$ ($\pm$ S.E.M.) granulocytes to plastic and $0.94 \pm 0.08 \times 10^6$ ($\pm$ S.E.M.) granulocytes to endothelial cells. The difference of adhesion to plastic and to endothelial cells appeared to increase with the number of washes (fig 1).

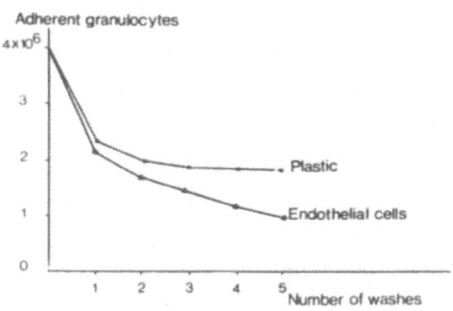

Figure 1. Adhesion of ^{51}Cr labelled granulocytes (4×10^6) from controls to Plastic Petri dishes and cultured endothelial cells. The curves represent the mean values of four duplicate experiments.

When the number of granulocytes added was increased the number of adhering leukocytes increased less to endothelial cells cultures than to plastic dishes. Adhesion was six times higher to plastic than to endothelial cells for the highest concentration of granulocytes added (32×10^6) (fig 2).

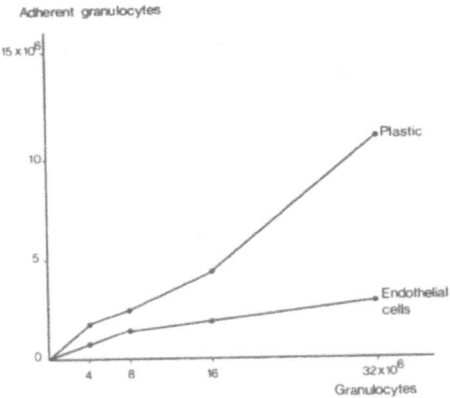

Figure 2. Concentration dependance of granulocytes adhesion
to plastic petri dishes and to cultured endothelial cells. Each point represents the number of
adhering cells after the fifth wash calculated
from the mean of ^{51}Cr counts for 3 duplicate experiments.

3.2. Adhesion of human promyelocytic leukemia cells (HL 60)
to endothelial cells and to plastic.

HL 60 cells were cultured in presence of retinoic acid for
1 to 8 days. The differentiation induced by retinoic acid
was estimated on morphological assessment by a differential
count on Wright Giemsa Slide preparations. HL 60 cells pro-
gressivly became mature myeloid cells and after 8 days 95 %
of the cells were differentiated.

Table 1. :

INCUBATION TIME WITH RETINOIC ACID	PROMYELOCYTIC CELLS %	MATURE MYELOID CELLS %	ADHESION TO PLASTIC %	ADHESION TO ENDOTHELIAL CELLS %
None	90	10	7.7	5.8
1 day	87	13	13.7	8.0
2 days	85	15	15.7	11.5
3 days	38	62	16.8	15.7
4 days	38	62	31.5	26.6
8 days	5	95	43.0	31.6

The uninduced HL 60 cells adhered poorly either to plastic
or to endothelial cells : 7.7 % (0.28 x 10^6) and 5.8 %

(0.24×10^6).

Induced HL 60 cells (8 days) adhered as well as normal granulocytes to plastic (HL 60 cells 1.72×10^6, normal granulocytes $1.76 \pm 0.2 \times 10^6$) (Fig 3).

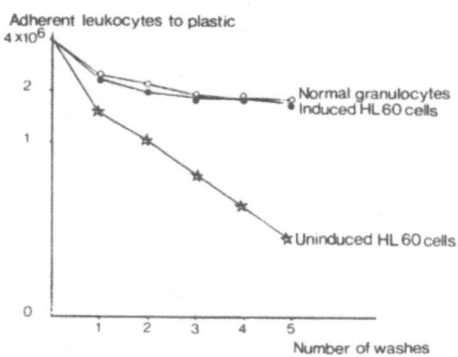

Figure 3. Adhesion of ^{51}Cr labelled HL 60 human promyelocytic leukemia cells (4×10^6) to Plastic Petri dishes.
Induced HL 60 cells were treated with retinoic acid for 8 days. Normal granulocytes adhesion is the mean of 4 duplicate experiments.

Adhesion of induced HL 60 cells to endothelial cells was slightly higher than that of normal granulocytes :
1.24×10^6 for HL 60 cells (8 days) $0.94 \pm 0.08 \times 10^6$ normal granulocytes (Fig 4).

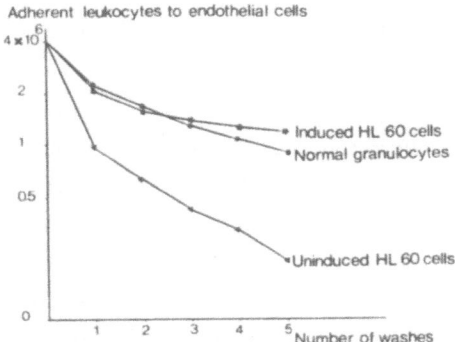

Figure 4. Adhesion of ^{51}Cr labelled HL 60 human promyelocytic leukemia cells (4 x 10^6) to endothelial cells. Normal granulocytes adhesion is the mean of 4 duplicate experiments.

4. DISCUSSION

The adhesion of normal isolated and unstimulated granulocytes to plastic estimated using a radiometric technique appears to be higher than to endothelial cells. This result seems different from those obtained after one wash by MAC GREGOR et al (3, 4) who found 4 % adhesion to plastic and 13 % to 26 % adhesion to endothelial cells. These differences could be explained by the fact that MAC GREGOR used non confluent endothelial cells, whole blood and an optical counting technique of non adhering leukocytes. Some variations in adhesion to plastic could also be due to the use of a different brand of plastic Petri dishes.

In addition, presence of serum proteins in the medium or absorbed on the surfaces tested can modify adhesion of leukocytes. BEESLEY et al (5) showed that the adhesion to glass was reduced by the presence of serum proteins.

Our results are comparable with those obtained by HOOVER et

al (6) who found after one wash 54 % adhering leukocytes to
plastic and 60 % to endothelial cells. After one wash we observed that 59 % of leukocytes adhered to plastic and 57 %
to endothelial cells. Other authors (7, 8) studying adhesion
of isolated leukocytes to endothelial cells found a percentage of adhering granulocytes after one wash varying between
44 and 46 %.

The technique using several washes and the counting of radioactivity in each wash possibly enhanced the sensitivity and
amplified the difference of adhesion to various surfaces.
The study of the development of adhesive properties of granulocytes precursors at different stages of maturation is
difficult to realize in man. The induced differentiation of
human promyelocytic leukemia cells (HL 60) permitted an in
vitro approach of this phenomenon. The HL 60, cells derived
from a patient with acute promyelocytic leukemia, proliferate continuously in suspension culture and consist of promye-
locytes (90 %) (9). Morphological changes can be induced by
incubation with butyrate, hypoxanthine, actinomycine D, di-
methyl sulfoxide (10) and retinoic acid (11) and these changes mimic normal myeloid differentiation. Induced HL 60
cells have also functionnal characteristics of normal peripheral blood leukocytes such as response to chemoattractants
(12, 13) and development of complement receptors. Furthermore COLLINS (12) showed that HL 60 cells induced with dime-
thyl sulfoxide have an increased percentage of complement
receptors than normal granulocytes.

The adhesion of HL 60 cells progressively increased during
induced maturation by retinoic acid. After 8 days, these
cells exhibited adhesive properties to plastic comparable to
those of normal granulocytes. The adhesion to endothelial
cells is also developed during induced maturation. After 8
days, when 95 % of the HL 60 cells were differentiated into
mature myeloid cells, adhesion to endothelial cells appears
to be better than adhesion of normal granulocytes isolated
from blood. The increased adhesive properties of induced

HL 60 cells may be a characteristic of young granulocytes or of abnormal leukocytes. The technique used in this work seems appropriate to study adhesion of granulocytes in human pathology.

ACKNOWLEDGEMENTS.

This work was supported by the grant Zedet of the Association Claude Bernard.

REFERENCES

1. Gallin J.I., Clark R.A., Kimball H.R. : Granulocyte chemotaxis an improved in vitro assay employing Cr^{51} labelled granulocytes. J. Immunol 1973, 110, 233-240.
2. Jaffe E.A., Nachman R.L., Becker G.G., Minick C.R. : Culture of human endothelial cells derived from umbilical veins : identification by morphologic and immunologic criteria. J. Clin. Invest. 1973, 52, 2745-2756.
3. Mac Gregor R.R., Macarak E.J., Kefalides N. : Comparative adherence of granulocytes to endothelial mololayers and nylon fiber. J. Clin. Invest. 1978, 61, 697-707.
4. Mac Gregor R.R., Friedman H.M., Macarak E.J., Kefalides N.A. : Virus infection of endothelial cells increases granulocyte adherence. J. Clin. Invest. 1980, 65, 1469-1477.
5. Beesley J.E., Pearson J.D., Carleton J.S., Hutchings A., Gordon J.L. : Interaction of leukocytes with vascular cells in culture. J. Cell. Sci. 1978, 33, 85-101.
6. Hoover R.L., Briggs R.T., Karnovsky M.J. : The adhesive interaction between polymorphonuclear leukocytes and endothelial cells in vitro. Cell 1978, 14, 423-428.
7. Boxer L.A., Allen J.M., Baehner R.L. : Diminished polymorphonuclear leukocyte adherence. J. Clin. Invest. 1980, 66, 268-274.
8. Oseas R., Hsin-Hsin Yang, Baehner R.L., Boxer L.A.: Lactoferrin : a promoter of polymorphonuclear leukocyte adhesiveness. Blood 1981, 57, 939-945.
9. Collins S.J., Gallo R.C., Gallgher R.E. : Continuous growth and differentiation of human myeloid leukemic cells in suspension culture. Nature 1977, 270, 347-349.
10. Collins S.J., Bodner A., Ting R., Gallo R.C. : Induction of morphological and functional differentiation of human promyelocytic leukemia cells (HL 60) by compounds which induce differentiation of murine leukemia cells. Int. J. Cancer 1980, 25, 213-218.
11. Breitman T.R., Selonick S.E., Collins S.J. : Induction of differentiation of the human promyelocytic leukemia cell line (HL 60) by retinoic acid. Proc. Natl. Acad. Sci. U S A 1980, 77, 2936-2940.
12. Collins S.J., Ruscetti F.N., Gallagher R.E., Gallo R.C. : Normal functional characteristics of cultured human promyelocytic leukemia cells (HL 60) after induction of dif--ferentiation by dimethylsulfoxide. J. Exp. Med. 1979, 149, 969-974.

13. Fontana J.A., Wright D.G., Schiffman E., Corcoran B.A.,
    Deisseroth A.B.: Development of chemotactic responsive-
    ness in myeloid precursor cells : studies with a human
    leukemia cell line. Proc.Natl. Acad. Sci. USA, 1980, 77,
    3664-3668.

IN VITRO METHODS FOR QUANTIFICATION OF GRANULOCYTE ADHESIVENESS
(COMMENTARY)

Jörg FEHR

As it is the case for the measurement of chemotaxis, in vitro
quantification of granulocyte adhesiveness is far from being
standardised, and we can be sure that there is still a long way
to go until we arrive at a method that will find broad acceptance
and that will produce comparable results when performed in different laboratories. The two studies to be commented on performed
by G.HOPEN (A) and A.COURILLON et al.(B) represent such steps on
a rather stony way.

Ad A: HOPEN correctly points out that we have to discriminate
between two different types of cellular adhesiveness to non-
biologic surfaces. Using a protein-free physiologic suspension
medium, there is apparently a direct adsorption of cells onto the
substratum which is passive, i.e.independent of the viability or
metabolic state of the cells. However, if proteins are added to
the suspension medium, they are rapidly adsorbed to the surface
and, in this case, adherence of cells occurs to such proteins;
researchers working on cell culture conditions have told us that
such an attachment represents an active process, i.e. dependent
on cell integrity and metabolic activity (1).As far as the passive
mechanism is concerned, it is certainly important to be aware of
it, but - at least from a biologic point of view - it has no relevance to the in vivo situation. Therefore, I strongly believe that
one should not consider protein/plasma as 'adhesion inhibitors'
but as compounds that provide the essential prerequisites to
overcome an artificial in vitro phenomenon. As an example, it is
known that in the absence of protein granulocytes do not move in
chemotactic in vitro devices.If protein is added (e.g.albumin),
the cells show spontaneous migratory capacity. Isn't it nonsense

to call then albumin a 'chemokinetic' factor just because it
allows the cell to overcome passive adsorption (paralysis)?

Although HOPEN deserves credit for bringing us to attention
the often neglected discrimination between active and passive cel
adherence, I believe that we cannot take it for granted that EDTA
is the ideal compound to dissect the two types of adhesion. EDTA
may not be an innocent divalent cation chelator but may also possess uncontrolled affinities to cell membranes, with subsequent
properties we do not know about yet. Furthermore, it may be pre-
mature and incorrect to assume close analogy between the mechanisms responsible for active adherence of granulocytes on the one
hand and surface attachment of fibroblasts and other tissue cells
on the other hand. As the anchoring apparatus of fibroblasts is
becoming unraveled these days, we are still far away from a definition of the structures that are responsible for granulocyte
attachment to surfaces.Our personal experience tells us that - as
soon as surface contact is reached and shear stresses are overcome
- firm granulocyte attachment occurs extremly rapidly. Another
point I have to draw attention to is the fact that the glass bead
system of HOPEN is apparently not able to pick up increased adhesiveness provoked by complement split products and other still
unknown stimulators in plasma of patients with inflammatory diseases (2), an observation that has been made by our group and
others as well. With respect to technical in vitro phenomena,I
have to mention that the interaction of non-biologic surfaces with
plasma proteins can result in the production of unexplained stimulators that do not reflect the in vivo situation. First, the
interaction of the complement system with cuprophane (cellophane)
(3) or nylon fibers (4) leads to activation of the system. Second,
nylon fibers and hydrophobic surfaces in general seem to adsorb
IgG in a way that the Fc portion becomes exposed to the medium
and granulocytes attach via their Fc receptors (5); therefore,
such assay systems cannot discriminate between intrinsic cellular
adhesiveness and secondarily induced in vitro immune adherence
via Fc receptors. Hence, the question remains if the assay systems presented allow for sufficient control and are appropriate
to pick up changes in granulocyte behaviour in physiology and

pathology.

Ad B: It is well understandable that the mentioned drawbacks
of the in vitro cellular adhesion assay systems have stimulated
the search for more physiologic methods. The study of COURILLON
et al. on the adhesion of granulocytes to cultured endothelial
cells represents such an example. Although such cellular monolayer surfaces promise to represent the physiologic situation
more closely, one has to admit that we have no proof that endothelial monolayers grown under in vitro conditions are indeed
identical to endothelial vessel linings. The influence of 'passive' and 'active' processes as well as protein interactions with
such biologic surfaces have not been studied at all up to the
present time. Therefore, it is certainly meritorious when the authors address themselves to the better definition of methodical
problems such as the influence of the washing procedure and the
role of the amount of leukocytes added.With respect to the washing
procedure, such methodical details may be crucial if we try to
dissect low affinity adhesion that is a prerequisite for any
crawling motion from the high affinity adhesion that is responsible for cell trapping at the inflammatory focus (6). With respect to the observation that the amount of granulocytes adhering
to the endothelium seems to be rather independent of the number
of cells added, the data presented allow no definite conclusions;
morphologic/morphometric studies would be needed to elucidate e.g.
if we are dealing with a satturation phenomenon or if only a sub-
population of endothelial cells allows granulocytes to attach. On
the other hand, granulocytes can apparently influence the behaviour of each other; as an example, it has been shown that increasing the amount of granulocytes added to a chemotactic chamber
leads to potentiation of migration (7).

The study on the development of adhesive properties of granulocyte precursors at different stages of maturation represents
a first application of the author's system to an investigative
problem. Instead of using in vitro differentiation of a commercial
cell line (HL 60), we have used a different approach and have
studied adhesive properties of myelopoietic human bone marrow
precursors on the one hand, and the whole spectrum of myelo-

poietic cells in the blood of untreated patients with chronic myeloid leukemia on the other hand. By performing careful cell differentials on adhesive cells in our culture dish assay system, we came to the conclusion that the ability of myelopoietic cells to respond to a known potent adhesion stimulus (n-formyl-Met-Leu-Phe) is acquired at the stage of the metamyelocyte whereas younger cells did not adhere in significant amounts. These results not only confirm the present data on HL 60 cells but also demonstrate that, under appropriate conditions, the culture dish assay is a representative system to study certain aspects of granulocyte - endothelium interactions.

REFERENCES:

A. HOPEN,G.: In vitro measurement of leukocyte adhesiveness. This workshop.
B. COURILLON,A., WAUTIER,M.P., ABITA,J.P.,WAUTIER,J.L.: Adhesion of granulocytes to human cultured endothelial cells. This workshop.
1. GRINNELL,F. 1978. Int. Rev. Cytol. 53:65-144
2. HOPEN,G. 1980. Scand.J.Inf.Dis. 24:50
3. CRADDOCK,P.R., FEHR,J. 1977. J.Clin.Invest. 59:879
4. FEHR,J.,JACOB, H.S. 1977. J.Exp.Med. 146:641
5. FEHR,J., DAHINDEN,C. 1980. Clin. Res. 28:310
6. FEHR,J., DAHINDEN,C. 1979. J.Clin.Invest. 64:8
7. TAKEUCHI and PERSELLIN 1979. Am.J.Physiol. 236:C22

SUBSTRATUM ADHESION AND THE MOVEMENT OF NEUTROPHIL LEUCOCYTES

J.M. LACKIE & A.F. BROWN

Neutrophil leucocytes must move in order to leave the bone marrow and must adhere and migrate in order to leave the blood. Not only can neutrophils move through endothelium and tissue, but they do so with great facility. Indeed they might be considered one of the most invasive of cells and as such their locomotory behaviour is of particular interest.

One parameter often thought likely to be important in cell movement is the adhesive interaction with the substratum. Varying the adhesiveness of the substratum is known to affect the movement of fibroblasts (Gail & Boone 1970: Carter 1967) and it seems obvious that adhesion will be a pre-requisite for movement. What is less obvious is that this may apply only to locomotion over a planar surface and not necessarily to movement in a matrix: this is discussed more extensively elsewhere (Lackie 1982; Wilkinson, this volume).

In the context of inflammation there may also be effects on neutrophil adhesion which affect the migratory response. Chemotactic factors alter the adhesion of neutrophils in a complex time- and dose-dependent fashion, consistent with a role for such factors in enhancing margination, stimulating emigration, directing movement and trapping cells at an inflammatory focus. This has been discussed in greater detail elsewhere (Lackie & Smith 1980). Many workers have reported effects on adhesion correlated with movement (Keller 1981 for review), but our attempts to provide a more general statement about the interaction have met with little success. A possible reason for this and the implications for our understanding of neutrophil behaviour are the subject of this paper.

Forward movement of a cell requires some form of transient anchorage through which the rearward reaction upon the environment is transmitted. On a plane substratum anchorage will involve adhesion and without adhesion no movement is possible. Non-adherent drifting cells are often seen in time-lapse films, sometimes under circumstances in which we can be confident that they are alive (see later). Excessive adhesion also stops movement and cells fall into two categories in this respect. Some cells are extensively flattened and although ruffling actively at their margins the cell body never makes appreciable excursions; other cells are restrained only by terminal attachments which are, presumably, irreversible adhesions at the uropod. The 'tail' may be more than two cell diameters in length and in brief films these cells might appear motile - only prolonged observation reveals their anchorage.

Somewhere between these two extremes lies an adhesive interaction with the substratum which permits adequate traction and reversibility of the adhesion (permanence would lead to tethering). It is usually assumed that the rate of locomotion will be optimum at a particular level of adhesiveness and the simplest assumption would be of a symmetrical bell-shaped curve when the rate of individual cell movement is plotted against substratum adhesiveness. This assumption is usually extended to the population and herein lies the major problem.

Increasing concentrations of bovine serum albumin (BSA) decrease the adhesiveness of rabbit neutrophils and as adhesion decreases so speed increases. Beyond a certain level, however, the speed begins to decrease, lending support to the idea of a population optimum (Lackie & Smith 1980). Another supporting observation comes from time-lapse studies in which the cells are moving on an inverted coverslip. Cells which fall off are, when retrospectively analysed, moving faster than the cells which remain attached (Lackie 1982).

If, however, we put neutrophils on substrata of very low adhesiveness, much lower than can be achieved with albumin, then we find that the rate of locomotion is more-or-less the same, although the proportion of motile cells is not (Table 1). The substrata in question are of glass coated with plasma fibronectin (Fn), gelatin or native collagen. The adhesive interaction with these surfaces, particularly collagen, is weak (or extremely short-lived, a possibility we cannot exclude) as shown in Figure 1. This may explain why endothelial monolayers are so much more adhesive for neutrophils than fibroblasts (Lackie & de Bono 1977) - endothelial cells do not have fibronectin on their luminal surfaces (Birdwell, Gospodarowicz & Nicolson 1978).

TABLE 1 . The movement of rabbit peritoneal exudate neutrophils on various substrata.

Glass coated with:	Adhesiveness[a] of substratum	No. & (%) motile cells	Speed ± s.d.[b] (µm/min)
1% BSA	High	16 (19)	6.3 ± 1.3
0.1% casein	Intermediate	15 (71)	7.1 ± 1.7
1% gelatin	Intermediate	14 (39)	5.7 ± 1.5
1% gelatin + 100µg/ml Fn	Very low	4 (9)	7.3 ± 2.6

(a) Based on aggregation and adhesion-to-coverslip assays as described in Lackie & Smith (1980). Collagen substrata are so non-adhesive that we have never managed to film cells satisfactorily.

(b) Cells were filmed at a 10 sec lapse interval and the distance moved per 10 frames measured and averaged for at least 200 frames per cell. The standard deviation is inappropriate for non-normally distributed data such as this: Mann-Whitney U-tests reveal no significant differences.

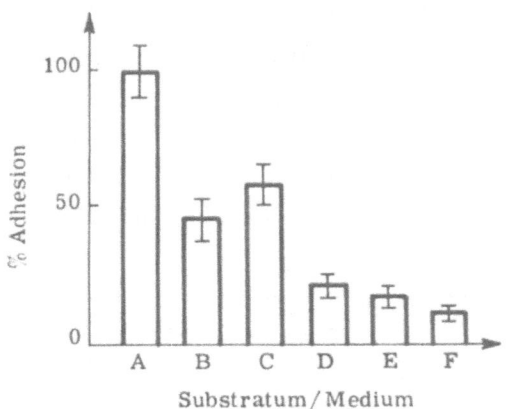

FIGURE 1   The adhesion of rabbit peritoneal neutrophils to various substrata relative to clean glass (100%). Cells were incubated for 30 min. at 37°C and non-adherent cells rinsed off. (a) Clean glass (b) 100µg/ml fibronectin (c) gelatin coated (d) gelatin + 100µg/ml fibronectin (e) collagen, and (f) collagen + fibronectin.

Thus, on surfaces of widely differing adhesiveness judged by the behaviour of cells in various sorts of adhesion assays, the locomotory rate of motile cells remains approximately constant. It should perhaps be remarked that immobility can arise in three ways, excessive adhesion, lack of adhesion and death. The dead cells are easily recognised and ignored but the other two are less easily distinguished and some subjective element is inevitable in interpreting films.

If we assess movement in another way, by the leading-front method in a micropore-filter assay, we find that verying the adhesion has no effect (Table 2).

TABLE 2   Movement in the rigid matrix of a micropore filter.   Rabbit neutrophils and fibronectin coated filters.

Concentration of Fn $\mu g/ml$	% adhesion ± s.d. (n)	Distance of leading front (μm) (n)
0	100 ± 3 (5)	36.9 ± 0.9 (4)
1	92 ± 6 (5)	41.6 ± 0.9 (4)
10	52 ± 5 (5)**	41.9 ± 1.0 (4)
100	33 ± 6 (3)**	41.4 ± 3.4 (4)

** p (no difference from control) < 0.001

Bovine fibronectin was prepared and used in adhesion assays as described by Brown & Lackie, 1981; 3µm pore filters were pre-soaked in fibronectin and the leading front measured (Zigmond & Hirsch 1973). Similar results were obtained with human blood neutrophils, with human and rabbit fibronectin in various combinations (Lackie, Brown & Allan, in preparation).

The absence of effect probably arises from the method, which assesses the movement of the fastest cells and disregards the population mobility. In some ways this is a virtue of the method, but the limitation must be recognised. Time-lapse methods, tedious though they are, give us more information. The range of locomotory rate is remarkable: in a series of film sequences a total of 93 rabbit neutrophils were tracked, each for an hour, in medium with 50% exudate fluid. The speed of an individual cell was fairly constant but there were cells moving at speeds between 2.2µm/min to 18.7µm/min with a population mean of 9.81 ± 3.4µm/min.

There are two ways in which the uniformity of speed on disparate substrata might be explained:

(i)   the adhesion optimum for movement is very broad,

(ii)   the expectation of a population optimum is wrong.

The former will not really explain the variability between the proportion of motile cells, drawn from the same population, on different substrata, whilst the latter is not obvious without further explanation. Because an important implication derives from this argument and because it has not, to our knowledge, been explicitly detailed elsewhere, we expand it below.

Suppose we are examining a population of cells with very different adhesive properties - but without knowing the exact distribution between classes of adhesiveness. We can arbitrarily define high, low and intermediate classes and might expect the proportions to vary from sample to sample, hence the variability in adhesiveness which is a major problem in comparing adhesion experiments (Lackie 1977). If we further *assume* that for each cell there is an optimum adhesiveness for locomotion and that all cells have potentially the same top speed, then:

(a) On a low-adhesion surface only the 'sticky' sub-population will move near their best speed and only some will move at top speed.

(b) On a highly-adhesive surface cells which gained no traction on the low-adhesive substratum of (a) will now move well but the remainder are stuck.

(c) On surfaces of intermediate adhesiveness the 'intermediate' class will be best adapted and there will be some cells from the 'high' and 'low' sub-classes which are moving sub-optimally.

Worked example to show the effect of varying the proportion of cells with particular adhesive properties.

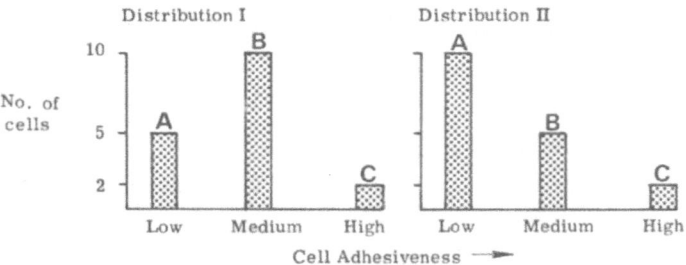

Assume : (1) cells at optimum 15μm/min
         (2) cells at sub-optimum 2μm/min
         (3) cells in the adjacent class respond sub-optimally.

Substratum adhesiveness	Optimal responders	Distribution	% motile	Mean speed μm/min (motile cells)
Low	(C)	I	70	4.2
Low	(C)	II	41	5.7
Intermediate	(B)	I	100	9.6
Intermediate	(B)	II	100	5.8
High	(A)	I	88	6.3
High	(A)	II	88	10.7

Notice that cells of distribution I seem to show a population optimum and that even if the same percentage are motile the speeds may vary.

Depending upon the *form* of the distribution of adhesive properties then the mean rate of locomotion will depend upon the proportion which are scored as motile - unless we are using a method such as the leading front method in which case the speed will be the same in all cases. (Variation in speed in the leading front method might be ascribed to effects on the motile machinery rather than on traction.)   On substrata which approach either of the extreme levels of adhesiveness the proportion of motile cells will be lower since only one tail of the distribution will contribute.

The idea that neutrophils are of widely differing adhesiveness is probably not unreasonable: in an aggregation assay many remain as single cells in suspension while others clump to doublets,   triplets and so on,   while yet others stick to the walls of the vessel.   Inverting a coverslip on which cells have been allowed to settle leads to a different proportion dropping off on different days and the proportion of anchored cells in film sequences varies markedly under supposedly identical conditions.   If the assumption of an optimum for adhesion for the individual cell is correct and the variability in the population is as we suppose then no 'population' optimum can be reproducibly detected by the sorts of assays we have attempted to use for this purpose.

The theoretical exercise which we have used to explain our failure to find a population optimum can easily be made more complicated by making more realistic assumptions - that top speeds are variable, that rate/adhesion curves are asymmetrical, that cells can move from sub-class to sub-class and so on.   In a sense we are frustrated in our experiments by an excellent design feature of the neutrophil.   There seem to be cells capable of responding well under a wide range of conditions. Had there been a single optimum level of adhesiveness for rapid locomotion for all cells in the population then we would have to suppose that the adhesive properties of connective tissue in different sites were very similar and relatively invariable under conditions of inflammatory stress, however caused.   By having an effector cell population of diverse behavioural capacity these design constraints on other tissues would be removed.

Summary

On substrata of widely differing adhesiveness the rate of movement of neutrophil leucocytes seems approximately constant although the proportion of motile cells varies.   It is suggested that this arises because of variability of adhesiveness of leucocytes within the population such that, at most levels of substratum adhesiveness, there are cells capable of normal movement. The idea that there is an optimum level of adhesiveness for the population as a whole is disputed and the possible utility of population diversity argued as justification.

Acknowledgement

This work was supported by an MRC project grant and MRC research studentship. We are grateful to Dr. R.B. Allan for the filter experiment described in Table 2.

References

Birdwell, C.R., Gospodarowicz, D. & Nicolson, G. (1978) Identification, localization and role of fibronectin in cultured bovine endothelial cells. *Proc, Nat. Acad. USA, 75,* 3273-7.

Brown, A.F. & Lackie, J.M. (1981) Fibronectin and collagen inhibit cell-substratum adhesion of neutrophil granulocytes. *Exp.Cell Res. 136,*225-3L

Carter, S.B. (1967) Haptotaxis and the mechanism of cell motility. *Nature (Lond) 213,* 256-60.

Gail, M.H. & Boone, C.W. (1970) The locomotion of mouse fibroblasts in tissue culture. *Biophys. J. 10,* 980-93.

Keller, H.U. (1981) The relationship between leucocyte adhesion to solid substrata, locomotion, chemokinesis and chemotaxis. In *Biology of the Chemotactic Response,* ed. Lackie, J.M. & Wilkinson, P.C. CUP, Cambridge.

Lackie, J.M. (1977) The aggregation of rabbit polymorphonuclear leucocytes (PMNs). Effects of agents which affect the acute inflammatory response and correlation with secretory activity. *Inflammation 2,* 1-15.

Lackie, J.M. (1982) Aspects of the behaviour of neutrophil leucocytes. In *The Social Behaviour of Cells,* ed. Curtis, A.S.G., Bellairs, R. & Dunn, G. pp.319-347. CUP, Cambridge.

Lackie, J.M. & de Bono, D. (1977) Interactions of neutrophil granulocytes (PMNs) and endothelium *in vitro. Microvascular Research 13,* 107-112.

Lackie, J.M. & Smith, R.P.C. (1980) Interactions of leucocytes and endothelium. In *Cell Adhesion and Motility,* ed. Curtis, A.S.G. & Pitts, J.D., CUP Cambridge.

Zigmond, S.H. & Hirsch, J.G. (1980) Leucocyte locomotion and chemotaxis. New methods for evaluation and demonstration of cell-derived chemotactic factor. *J. Exp. Med. 137,* 187-410.

THE ROLE OF BLOOD FLOW IN THE DISTRIBUTION OF LYMPHOCYTES AND LYMPHOBLASTS IN VIVO

C.A. OTTAWAY and D.M.V.PARROTT

The migration of lymphoid cells from one tissue to another facilitates the initiation and expression of immune responses in vivo. Investigations of this lymphoid cell traffic most frequently consist of assessing the distribution of isotopically labelled lymphoid cells from a donor animal at a single time point (usually 18-24 h) after their intravenous injection into a compatible recipient. In such experiments the transferred cells are not distributed uniformly throughout the recipient's tissues and observations show that different types of lymphoid cells have a propensity to accumulate in some tissues more readily than others.

Lymphoid cell traffic to the non-lymphoid small intestine, Peyer's patches and mesenteric lymph nodes is a useful experimental model of the selective localization of different cell populations. It has long been recognized that small lymphocytes can be found in large numbers in Peyer's patches and the mesenteric lymph nodes 18-24 h after transfer, but few can be identified within the intestinal mucosa (1). These basic findings have been confirmed in a number of species and are in strong contrast to the behaviour of lymphoblasts from the mesenteric nodes, thoracic duct lymph or intestinal lymph which accumulate readily in the intestinal mucosa (1-6), but do not accumulate in mesenteric lymph nodes to the same extent as small lymphocytes (7, 8). Lymphoblasts from subcutaneous lymph nodes however are limited in their ability to accumulate in the intestine (6, 7), although they readily accumulate in inflamed skin or the peritoneal cavity (9). This selective localization of lymphoid cells, commonly referred to as homing, has led to the view that migrating cells somehow discriminate between different tissue destinations during their intravascular journey. Different cell populations have been attributed with the ability to seek out particular tissues. For example, it has been inferred that only lymphoblasts generated in the lymphoid tissues serving the mucosa are able to gain entry to the small intestine whereas peripheral blast cells or small lymphocytes are somehow excluded. The extent to which selective migration is determined by the local presence of antigen, the properties of the lymphoid cells themselves and organ specific factors are currently important but largely unresolved questions. We have been investigating the feasibility of interpreting the kinetics of lymphoid cell accumulation in tissues as a means of addressing these questions as well as investigating the role of the delivery of cells to tissues by the blood stream.

KINETICS OF ACCUMULATION:

For a transferred labelled cell to be found in a particular tissue, the cell must arrive in the appropriate vascular bed, attach to and cross the endothelium, and stay in the tissue long enough to be found. Although each of these processes is very complex and influenced by many factors, we chose to make the following assumptions; first, that the rate of lymphoid cell uptake into a tissue is directly proportional to the number of cells delivered randomly by the blood stream and second, that the rate of cell loss from the tissue is directly proportional to the number of those cells present in the tissue (10).

Under these circumstances, the number of labelled cells present in the tissue 0 at any given time can be described (10) as

$$n_\theta(t) = k_\theta \ e^{-\lambda_\theta t} \int_0^t f_\theta(t) \ CO(t) \ n_b(t) \ e^{\lambda_\theta t} \ dt + n_o \ e^{-\lambda_\theta t} \qquad (1)$$

where $n_\theta t$ is the number of labelled cells in the tissue, k_θ is the proportion of cells delivered by the blood stream that is taken up by that tissue, λ_θ is the proportion of the labelled cells in the tissue which is lost per unit time, $f_\theta(t)$ is the fraction of the cardiac output, $CO(t)$, which goes to the tissue, $n_b(t)$ is the concentration of labelled cells in the blood, and n_o is the number of labelled cells in the tissue at the start of the time period considered.

When the concentration of labelled cells in the blood can be approximated by a simple relationship, Eqn 1 simplifies (10). For example, if the concentration of labelled cells in the blood is constant $(n_b(t)=B)$, and the blood flow to the tissue is assumed to be stable, then Eqn 1 becomes

$$n_\theta(t) = k_\theta \ \bar{f}_\theta \ \overline{CO} \ \frac{B}{\lambda_\theta} \ (1 - e^{-\lambda_\theta t}) + n_o e^{-\lambda_\theta t} \qquad (2)$$

A series of observations during such a time period can then be used to solve for the unknowns k_θ and λ_θ when the blood flow to the tissue is known. For convenience, λ_θ can be expressed as a half time where $T\frac{1}{2} = \ln 2 / \lambda$

The time course of accumulation of lymphoblasts in the small intestine (Fig 1) and thoracic duct lymphocytes in the mesenteric lymph node (fig 2) are amenable to interpretation using this simple model. Furthermore, estimates of the kinetic parameters (k and λ) derived from observations over limited time periods provide a reasonable approximation of the time course which is observed throughout the 24 h after cell transfer (Fig 1, 2). Examination of the accumulation of various lymphoid cell populations in mice and rats suggest that the uptake of lymphocytes and lymphoblasts into mesenteric lymph nodes and Peyer's patches is about an order of magnitude greater than their uptake into the small intestine (Table I and II). Unexpectedly, the results show that lymphoblasts are taken up by mesenteric nodes with approximately the same efficiency as small lymphocytes. The loss of small lymphocytes from the node, however, is slower than that of lymphoblasts.

For the small intestine, the uptake of small lymphocytes was found to be of the same order of magnitude as that for different lymphoblast populations. Here, however, only mesenteric

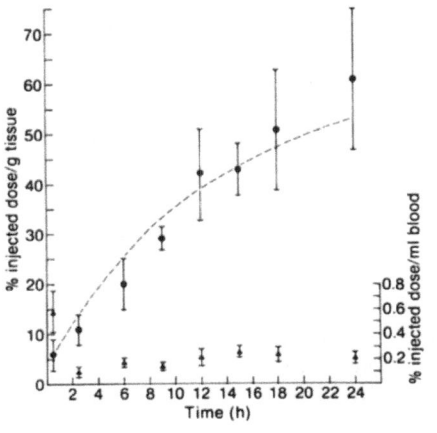

Fig. 1:
Accumulation of ^{51}Cr-TDL in rat mesenteric lymph nodes. The amount of injected radioactivity in mesenteric node/g (●) and blood/ml (△) (means±S.D.) as reported by Smith and coworkers (8) for different times after cell transfer was analysed. Estimates of k=0.22 for the fraction of delivered cells extracted from the blood and λ =0.08h^{-1} for the loss of cells from the node were obtained from the observations between 6 and 15h. Using these values, the expected accumulation (---) was calculated from equation 2 starting with the 0.5h observation and assuming a constant blood level of 0.2%/ml.

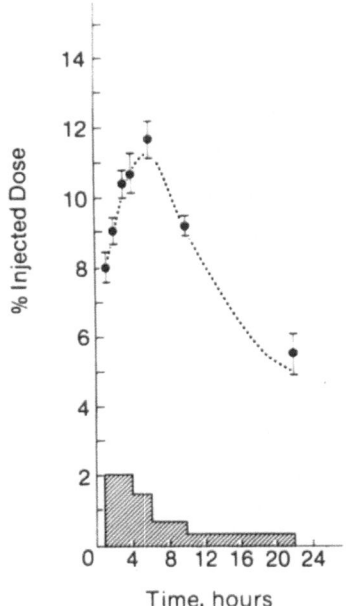

Fig. 2:
Accumulation of ^{125}I-UdR-MLN lymphoblasts in the small intestine of the mouse (●) (mean±sem). The hatched area represents the radioactivity found per ml of blood at various times after cell transfer. The observations over the first 4h were analyzed and gave estimates of k=0.01 for the uptake of cells and λ =0.11h^{-1} for the loss of cells from the tissue. Using these values, the accumulation expected for the entire experiment was calculated from equation 2 starting with the 1h observation.

Table 1.   Results of the analysis of the accumulation of lymphoid cells in mesenteric lymph nodes.

Recipient	Cells transferred	k	$T\frac{1}{2}$ (hours)
Mouse	^{51}Cr-MLN	0.23	1.7
"	^{51}Cr-PLN*	0.29	5.8
"	^{51}Cr-(MLN+PLN)*	0.24	7.7
"	^{125}I-UdR-MLN	0.18	0.2
"	^{125}I-UdR-PLN	0.20	0.6
Rat	^{51}Cr-TDL	0.22	8.7

Cells from mesenteric lymph nodes (MLN) and/or peripheral nodes (PLN) or thoracic duct lymph (TDL) were labelled with ^{51}Cr or ^{125}I-UdR in vitro.   Cell populations enriched for T cells by passage through nylon-wool columns designated *

k,   the proportion of delivered cells which are taken up by tissue.
$T\frac{1}{2}$,   the half-time for cells in the tissue ($T\frac{1}{2} = \ln2/\lambda$)
The results for rat MLN obtained from analysis of published observations (8).

Table II.   Results of the analysis of the accumulation of lymphoid cells in the small intestine.

Recipient	Cells transferred	k	$T\frac{1}{2}$(hours)
Mouse	^{51}Cr-MLN	0.01	0.9
"	^{51}Cr-PLN	0.01	0.7
"	^{51}Cr-(MLN+PLN)*	0.01	0.6
"	^{125}I-UdR-MLN	0.01	3.1
"	^{125}I-UdR-PLN	0.02	0.6
"	^{125}I-UdR-MLN†	0.01	6.3
" (Peyer's patch)	^{125}I-UdR-MLN	0.11	0.7
Rat	^{51}Cr-TDL†	0.01	2.1
" (Peyer's patch)	^{51}Cr-TDL	0.17	2.5

† Small intestine without Peyer's patch tissue, in other experiments small intestine left intact.
k, $T\frac{1}{2}$ and cell populations as in Table 1.

lymphoblasts were likely to be retained for long periods of time and the other cell populations were lost rapidly from the intestine (Table II).

The preferential localization of these cell populations observed 18-24 h after cell transfer in different tissues is therefore predominantly the result of selective retention of arriving cells.

RELATIONSHIPS TO BLOOD FLOW:

The pattern of lymphoid cell localization within certain tissues directly reflects regional differences in the delivery of blood flow. In the normal small intestine, the localization of mesenteric lymphoblasts is not even along the small bowel. In experiments designed to assess how the localization of mesenteric lymphoblasts in the small intestine might be related to their delivery to particular regions of the small intestine, we found that there was a gradient of regional blood flow along the small intestine (11). When the fractional distribution of the cardiac output was measured using the indicator ^{86}RbCl in animals that had received lymphoblasts at 1, 4, 6, 18 or 24 h previously, there was a strong correlation between the lymphoblast accumulation and the delivery of blood flow to particular regions of the small intestine (11). This was so regardless of the time after cell transfer at which the accumulation of blast cells and blood flow were assessed and lymphoblast populations from either mesenteric or peripheral lymph nodes showed a similar correlation to the delivery of blood along the small intestine in spite of variations in their ability to accumulate in the gut (11).

The correlation of localization with the distribution of blood flow implies that the way in which a given population interacts with the normal small intestine is more or less uniform throughout the small intestine, and that regional differences in accumulation can be a direct result from regional differences in delivery. Indeed, when animals were raised on an elemental diet containing no macromolecular materials, the same delivery dependent behaviour of mesenteric lymphoblast accumulation was observed (12). Lymphoblast localization within the small intestine of mice fed the elemental diet was altered compared with pellet fed mice, but only in the distal small intestine where there was a significant reduction in the fraction of the cardiac output received by the tissue (12).

The distribution of small lymphocytes within recipients shows a different relationship to blood flow. The lymphoid organs of mice receive a lower specific perfusion than tissues such as the intestine and, although lymph nodes in different parts of the body vary in size, their regional blood flow is proportional to their weight (13). When the localization of ^{51}Cr labelled nodal lymphocytes within different lymph nodes was assessed 24 h after cell transfer in conjunction with the distribution of ^{86}RbCl, there was a significant correlation between the localization of the labelled cells and the blood flow to lymph nodes throughout the body (13). The probability of finding a particular transferred lymphocyte within a given node appears to be directly related to the perfusion of the node and suggests that the processes controlling the uptake and retention of these cells is similar in various lymph nodes.

ALTERATIONS WITH ANTIGENIC STIMULATION:

Stimulated lymph nodes reacting to various antigens undergo proliferation and there is an increase in the number of lymphocytes entering or leaving the node (14, 15). When mice are presented with an increased antigenic load in the form of an enteric infection with the nematode Trichinella spiralis, the fraction of the cardiac output delivered to the mesenteric lymph nodes is increased, but that to Peyer's patches is not (Fig 3). The increased blood flow to the mesenteric nodes is proportional to their increased weight (Fig 4), and similar blood flow changes related to the altered mass of stimulated nodes have been identified in rabbits (16), sheep (17) and mice (13) responding to simpler antigens.

This expansion of regional blood flow to a stimulated node may be an important physiological mechanism facilitating the increased delivery of cells to the challenged tissue. Increased lymphocyte

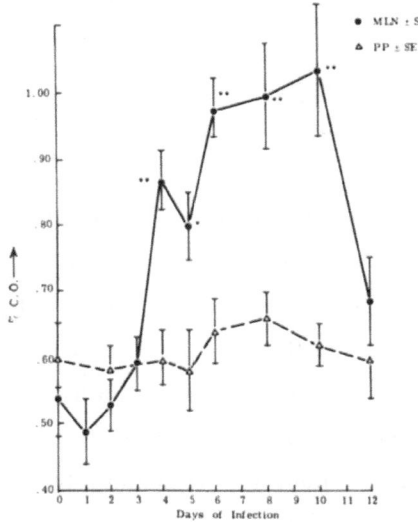

Fig. 3:
The regional blood flow
(% cardiac output determined with ^{86}RbCl) received
by gut lymphoid tissue and
mesenteric nodes at vari-
ous times after T.spiralis
infection. (Mean±S.D. for
4 mice per group).
* P<0.05 and ** P<0.01 for
comparison to uninfected
controls.

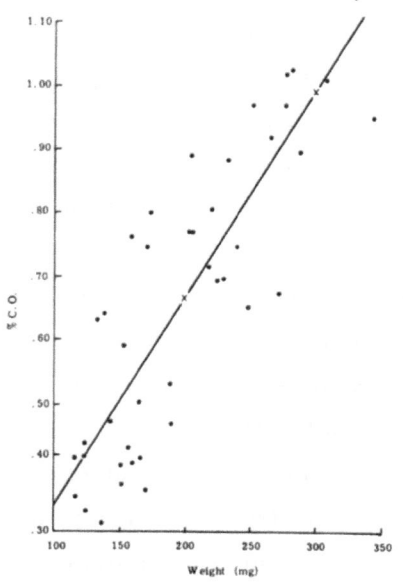

Fig. 4:
The relationship of the
fraction of the cardiac
output received and the
weight of mesenteric nodes
at different stages of infection with T.spiralis.
Regression analysis gave
a correlation coefficient
of 0.85, P<0.001.

traffic through stimulated nodes in sheep has been found to occur at the same time as increased blood flow to the node (17). In mice responding to skin application of contact sensitizers, there is an increased accumulation of transferred small lymphocytes in the subcutaneous lymph nodes which is directly proportional to the increased blood supply to the nodes (13).

How this altered delivery may affect the efficiency of extraction of cells by the lymph nodes has not yet been determined. The major difference in the efficiency with which lymphoid cells can be taken up by lymph nodes as opposed to non-lymphoid tissue (11) may be related to the specialized high endothelium of the post-capillary venules which has been recognized in some species (1). The microvasculature of lymph nodes is further specialized in that arterio-venous shunts leading to the high endothelial venules have been identified (18) and a substantial part of the hyperemia of lymph nodes may be the result of increased flow through these structures.

A number of observations suggest that the retention of cells can be affected by antigenic stimulation. The lymphocyte output in the efferent lymph of sheep nodes can decrease for a short time after the node is stimulated by certain antigens without alteration in lymph flow (14, 15). This reaction can occur even in the face of increased lymphocyte delivery to the node (15) and a similar reduction in the output of lymphocytes from the node can occur following the local activation of complement in unstimulated nodes (19).

Alteration in the retention of cells can also occur in non-lymphoid tissues. In the small intestine of mice undergoing infection with T. spiralis, there is an increase in the accumulation of mesenteric lymphoblasts compared to normal animals (20). Maximal enhancement of the localization of lymphoblasts occurs early in the infection, prior to the development of increased blood flow (20), altered vascular permeability (9) or the appearance of morphological changes in the small intestine (21). Examination of the kinetics of accumulation of mesenteric lymphoblasts in the small intestine of infected mice suggests that the enhanced accumulation of blast cells is the result of altered retention of cells within the mucosa rather than a change in their recruitment from the blood stream (22).

These studies suggest that many of the alterations of lymphoid cell traffic which occur during antigenic stimulation may result from changes in the delivery of cells to tissues combined with mechanisms which allow the selective retention of admitted cells after their arrival within the tissues. No experimental evidence is available at present to show that the extraction of cells by tissues changes with antigenic stimulation. Most of our present knowledge about lymphoid cell migration is based on observations at late times after cell transfer. We suggest that interpretation of the kinetics of cell accumulation in conjunction with measurements of the delivery of blood borne cells can provide detailed information about the migration process and will be helpful in dissecting the contribution of antigenic events to alterations in cell migration.

This work was supported by the Medical Research Council of Canada (MA7393) and the United Kingdom (G8011059).

REFERENCES
1. Gowans JL and Knight EJ, 1964. Proc. R. Soc. B. 159 257
2. Hall JG, Parry DM and Smith ME, 1972. Cell Tiss. Kinet. 5 269
3. Guy-Grand D, Griscelli C and Vassalli P, 1974. Europ. J. Immunol. 4 435
4. Parrott DMV and Ferguson A, 1974. Immunology 26 571
5. McWilliams M, Phillips-Quagliata JM and Lamm ME, 1975. J. Immunol. 115 54
6. Hall JG, Hopkins J and Orlans E, 1977. Europ. J. Immunol. 7 30
7. Rose ML, Parrott DMV and Bruce RG, 1976. Immunology 31 723
8. Smith ME, Martin AF and Ford WL, 1980. Monogr. Allergy 16 203
9. Rose ML, Parrott DMV and Bruce RG, 1976. Cell Immunol 27 36
10. Ottaway CA and Parrott DMV, 1981. Immunology Lettr. 2 283
11. Ottaway CA and Parrott DMV, 1980. Immunology 41 955
12. Ottaway CA and Parrott DMV, 1981. Gut 22 376

144

13. Ottaway CA and Parrott DMV, 1979   J exp. Med. 150 218
14. Hall JG and Morris B, 1965.   J. exp. Med. 121 901
15. Cahill RNP, Frost H and Trnka Z, 1976.   J. exp. Med,
        143 870
16. Herman PG, Lyonnet D, Fingerhut F and Tuttle RN, 1976)
        Lymphology 9 101
17. Hay JB and Hobbs BB, 1977.   J. exp. Med. 145 31
18. Herman PG, Utsunomiya R and Hessel SJ, 1979.
        Immunolgy 36 793
19. McConnel I, Hopkins J and Lachmann P, 1980. in "Blood
        Cells and Vessel Walls: Functional Interactions",
        Ciba Foundation Symp. No. 71, 167, Excerpta Medica,
        Amsterdam.
20. Ottaway CA, Manson-Smith DF, Bruce RG and Parrott DMV,
        1980.   Immunology 41 963
21. Manson-Smith DF, Bruce RG and Parrott DMV, 1979
        Cell. Immunol. 47 285
22. Ottaway CA, Bruce RG, Manson-Smith DF and Parrott DMV,
        1981.   Submitted.

LOCOMOTION AND ADHESION OF NEUTROPHILS AND THE ROLE OF BLOOD FLOW IN LYMPHOCYTE MIGRATIONS: COMMENTARY.

P. C. WILKINSON

There are really two separate problems arising from these papers and I shall discuss them separately. Firstly, Dr. Lackie discusses the relationship between adhesion and locomotion of neutrophil leukocytes and whether our experiments provide a realistic approach to this relationship. Secondly Drs. Ottaway and Parrott discuss what factors are involved in the accumulation of lymphocytes in tissues in vivo and suggest that changes in blood flow are of major importance.

Adhesion and locomotion. During recent years there have been high hopes that the availability both of adhesion assays and of assays for locomotion and chemotaxis would allow some generalizations to be made about the relationship between the two, and about adhesion optima for leukocyte locomotion. One of the particular hopes was that the increased attachment of circulating leukocytes to the vascular endothelium at a site of inflammation might be explained if contact with chemotactic factors made the leukocytes stickier. The idea that chemotactic factors did make neutrophil leukocytes sticky was supported by the finding that these factors induce a rapid and transient rise in cell-cell aggregation (1, 2). However, noone has shown, partly perhaps for technical reasons, that this is accompanied by a chemotactic-factor-induced increase in leukocyte-to-endothelium adhesiveness. From the interesting findings presented by Dr. Fehr to this meeting, it now seems likely that the aggregation assay does not parallel adhesion assays of other types, thus we cannot generalize that if a leukocyte

becomes stickier for other leukocytes, it is necessarily also more
adhesive for other surfaces. This is not altogether surprising since
adhesiveness is not an absolute property of a cell but an expression of
the interaction between the cell and the surface with which it comes
into contact, and this interaction will be different for each surface that
is studied, a point that is also implicit in Dr. Lackie's paper. We
still lack evidence that chemotactic factors are involved in the attachment of leukocytes to endothelia and in their migration across endothelia.

The main thrust of Dr. Lackie's paper was to suggest that any
population of neutrophils is heterogeneous in respect to adhesion,
thus no generalization can be made about the adhesiveness of the whole
population. If this is true it means that the information given by the
adhesion assays presently available is limited, because most of these
depend on measuring the adhesiveness of cell populations; and that
progress in understanding the locomotion:adhesion relationship is likely
to be poor until we get better adhesion assays. Certainly up to now
progress has been poor and the hopes mentioned at the beginning of this
commentary have not been fulfilled. However, as Dr. Lackie points
out, from the point of view of the leukocyte, if not from that of the
investigator, this heterogeneity is a good thing because, given a population of leukocytes whose adhesive properties vary widely moving on a
variety of surfaces whose adhesive properties also vary widely, it is
very likely that, in any given circumstance, there are going to be some
leukocytes that find conditions favourable for locomotion. Thus a
cellular inflammatory response would be favoured irrespective of
possibly widely varying surface properties of the tissues of the body.
A homogeneous population of cells with fastidious adhesion requirements
would probably not be very successful as inflammatory cells.

Another focus of debate in the general area of cell adhesion, which
cropped up several times in discussion, was the possibility that leukocyte
chemotaxis is really a form of haptotaxis (3), i.e. that cells recognize

and move up adhesive gradients.   Prime requirements for such a theory are (a) that the chemotactic factors do bind to substrata and (b) that leukocytes recognize not only fluid-phase gradients but substratum-bound gradients.   Data presented in our own paper suggests that both (a) and (b) do, in fact, occur.   However, another requirement of the theory is that chemotactic factors increase cell adhesion in a dose-dependent manner, a requirement that is unlikely to be fulfilled if Dr. Lackie's findings on adhesion heterogeneity are correct.   The evidence at present does not support this idea, indeed there is evidence that chemotactic factors reduce cell adhesion (4).   There is now good evidence that many chemotactic responses are triggered by ligand-receptor coupling and that leukocytes possess a sensory mechanism that allows them to detect differences in ligand concentration across the cell diameter, even though the leukocytes are on surfaces that do not allow locomotion.   My own view is that effects of chemotactic factors on cell adhesion are probably of secondary importance:- providing a suitable environment for locomotion:- and that what the cell detects is not an adhesion gradient but a gradient of discrete ligands that bind (irrespective of adhesion conditions) to defined domains on the cell surface; - receptors if you will; - with lamellipodium formation being favoured in the direction of highest ligand concentration.

Lymphocytes.

The lymphocytes present unique problems to the student of locomotion and adhesion because they are highly motile and yet very poorly adhesive to most biological surfaces.   We have suggested here that this might be because they can use three-dimensional lattices for non-adhesive propulsion.   However, the poor adhesiveness of lymphocytes has retarded progress in devising assays to investigate their locomotor properties in vitro.   In particular the study of lymphocyte chemotaxis and other forms of directed locomotion lags a long way behind that of neutrophils, and chemotaxis in lymphocytes is still rather poorly

documented.   Despite the fact that it is still very difficult to demonstrate that chemotaxis of any cell-type occurs in vivo, most of us now
accept that chemotaxis is important for recruiting neutrophils into
inflammatory lesions because the evidence for the phenomenon from
in vitro work is so massive.   Lymphocytes (or particularly lymphoblasts and other immunologically-activated lymphoid cells) also migrate
into inflammatory lesions and chemotaxis may play some part in this,
but, in addition, they show many other forms of migration in vivo
including recirculation between blood and lymph and recruitment into
various non-lymphoid tissues such as the intestine.   These migrations
are carried out by populations of unactivated small lymphocytes,
concerning which there is very scanty evidence for chemotaxis or other
forms of directed locomotion.   Drs. Ottaway and Parrott present a
theoretical and experimental examination of the migration and accumulation of lymphocytes in normal tissues or immunologically-stimulated
tissues using the intestine and the mesenteric lymph nodes (which drain
the intestine) as models.   They show that the differential localization
of lymphoid cells to different regions of the intestine can be directly
accounted for by differences in blood flow to those regions, and that a
similar generalization can be made about localization to lymph nodes.
Thus there is no necessity to invoke the hypothesis that, at points of
high accumulation of lymphocytes, there is a specialized interaction of
lymphocytes with vascular endothelium or directed locomotion of
lymphocytes to those sites, to explain this differential localization.
This is also true of immunologically-activated sites.   Such sites
experience an increase in regional blood flow which is consistent with
and proportional to the increase in lymphocyte accumulation.   This
observation is of interest since it suggests that antigen-specific
chemotaxis may not be of major importance in recruiting lymphocytes
into sites of antigen deposition.   In vitro, lymphocytes from immun-
ologically primed animals do show chemotaxis towards the priming
antigen (5).   However, it is possible that this is a mechanism that

allows short-range recognition of antigen-bearing cells by lymphocytes already present in the lesion (such as may be required for cooperative immune reactions) rather than for recruitment of lymphocytes from the blood. In inflammatory lesions the local recruitment of lymphoblasts and activated lymphocytes may be different and may resemble more closely the recruitment of phagocytic cells into the same lesions (which is clearly due to chemically-directed locomotion), and it is probably no coincidence that chemotaxis of lymphoblasts can be shown more readily in vitro than chemotaxis of small lymphocytes. The problems with unravelling the locomotor properties of lymphocytes are exacerbated by the fact that lymphocytes are extremely heterogeneous, so that different populations may show quite different characteristics. However, the approach of Ottaway and Parrott has a valuable lesson, for a meeting devoted largely to the investigation of leukocyte behaviour in defined microenvironments, in reminding us that in the whole animal changes in blood flow can result in proportional changes in cellular distribution and that this, as well as the physical and chemical properties of the blood cells themselves, must be taken into account in the detailed description of the migratory behaviour of these cells.

REFERENCES

1. Craddock P R, Hammerschmidt D, White J G, Dalmasso A P and Jacob H S. 1977. J. clin. Invest. 60, 260-264.
2. O'Flaherty J T, Kreutzer D L and Ward P A. 1977. J. Immunol. 119, 232-239.
3. Carter S B. 1967. Nature, 208, 1183-1187
4. Smith R P C, Lackie J M and Wilkinson P C. 1979. Exp. Cell Res., 122, 169-177.
5. Wilkinson P C, Parrott D M V, Russell R J and Sless F. 1977. J. exp. Med., 145, 1158-1168.

INCREASED VASCULAR PERMEABILITY FOLLOWING INTERACTION BETWEEN POLYMORPHO-
NUCLEAR NEUTROPHILS AND VASCULAR ENDOTHELIAL CELLS

T.J. WILLIAMS

1. INTRODUCTION

During an inflammatory reaction the walls of microvessels,which normally
have a low permeability to macromolecules, become leaky to blood proteins.
The increased permeability to proteins upsets the hydrodynamic equilibrium
in the tissue resulting in fluid efflux from microvessels and, as a
consequence, tissue swelling.   These effects on the microvessel walls,
mainly on the post-capillary venules, together with the accompanying
increased blood flow due to arteriolar dilatation, are thought to be caused
by the release of chemicals in the tissue.   Another characteristic feature
of inflammation is the accumulation of white blood cells, predominantly
polymorphonuclear (PMN) neutrophils in the early stages.   This phenomenon
is also thought to be due to the release of chemicals, 'chemotactic factors'
produced in response to the inflammatory stimulus.

Analysis of a simple inflammatory model in skin has revealed a link
between the three features of inflammation discussed above. Firstly, oedema
formation is dependent on two factors: the magnitude of elevated
permeability of venules and the level of arteriolar dilatation (1,2).
These two factors can be controlled by two entirely different chemicals.
Secondly, by some unexplained mechanism PMN neutrophils are able to increase
venular permeability to plasma proteins (3).   Thus, certain chemicals
capable of causing PMN neutrophils to accumulate in a tissue, when in the
presence of a vasodilator substance, are very potent in inducing oedema
formation.   In fact, some of these chemotactic substances, for example,
the complement fragment C5a (4), although much more potent than classical
oedema-inducing substances such as histamine, when in the presence of a
potent vasodilator such as a prostaglandin (E_1,E_2 or I_2).

These observations may explain the frequent reports in the literature
that depletion of circulating white cells suppresses oedema formation in

different animal models.   Our experiments using combinations of chemotactic
substances and vasodilator prostaglandins show that protein leakage is
detectable within 5-6 minutes of intradermal injection (3).   By this time
it has been observed both by electronmicroscopy and by vital light
microscopy that there is a very close association between PMN neutrophils
and the endothelial cells of post capillary venules.   This interaction
between the leukocyte and the vessel wall may be a fundamental component of
the inflammatory response.

2. METHOD OF MEASURING OEDEMA FORMATION(5)

All experiments were carried out using male New Zealand White rabbits
(3.5 - 4 kg body weight).   Each animal was given an intravenous injection
of $^{131}I-$ or ^{125}I-human serum albumin followed by intradermal injections of
test materials in 0.1 ml volumes into the clipped dorsal skin.   Each
test sample was   given as   six replicate injections.   Thirty minutes
later, animals were killed using an intravenous barbiturate overdose, the
dorsal skin was removed and the injection sites punched out for counting
in an automatic gamma-counter.   The amount of plasma exudation in each
skin sample was expressed in terms of a volume of plasma by dividing each
sample count by the count obtained with 1 μl of blood plasma.

3. THE INVOLVEMENT OF PROSTAGLANDINS

The model used in these studies was the inflammatory reaction to intradermally-injected zymosan (yeast-cell walls) in the rabbit (5).   Non-
steroid anti-inflammatory compounds, which are known to inhibit prostaglandin
synthesis, suppressed oedema formation in this model (4).   This suppression
was reversed by local injections of vasodilator prostaglandins (PGE_1,PGE_2
or PGI_2) (4) in spite of the observation that prostaglandins alone were
not able to induce significant leakage of plasma proteins (1,2).   Thus,
it was deduced that the oedema response to zymosan was produced by two
mediators acting synergistically: a vasodilator prostaglandin and an
unknown permeability-increasing substance (see Fig.1) (2).

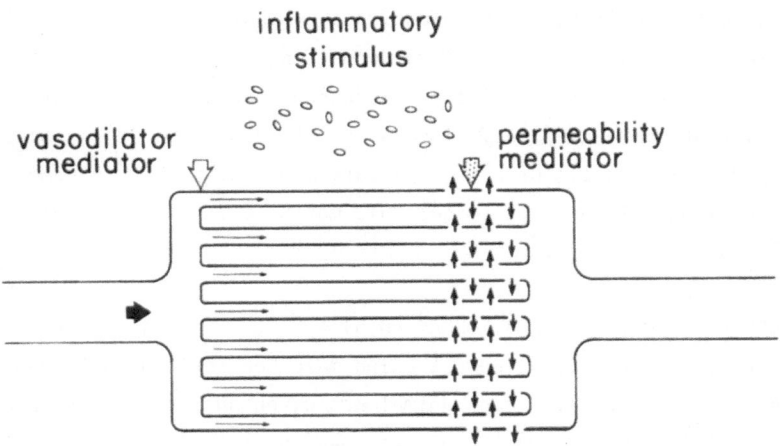

inflammatory
stimulus

vasodilator
mediator

permeability
mediator

"The Two Mediator Hypothesis", Williams & Peck,
Nature. 270 : 215 (1977)

FIGURE 1. A diagrammatic representation of the skin microvascular
bed. In response to a microbial stimulus two chemicals are
released which produce oedema by synergism: a prostaglandin acts
on arterioles to induce dilatation; another substance increases
venular permeability to macromolecules.

4. THE INVOLVEMENT OF COMPLEMENT

Histamine antagonists and inhibitors of kinin formation had no effect on
oedema formation in the model (4). For this reason we decided to investigate if an unknown permeability-increasing mediator could be generated in
tissue fluid in the presence of zymosan. Zymosan was incubated with blood
plasma or lymph, the zymosan was then removed by centrifugation and the
fluid tested in rabbit skin. Figure 2 shows the results of such an
experiment. It was clear that plasma incubated with zymosan was able to
induce oedema formation, but only if a vasodilator substance was added
(PGE_1 in this experiment) (4).

Subsequently, it has been shown that the active component generated in
plasma is C5a, a fragment of the fifth component of complement (4).

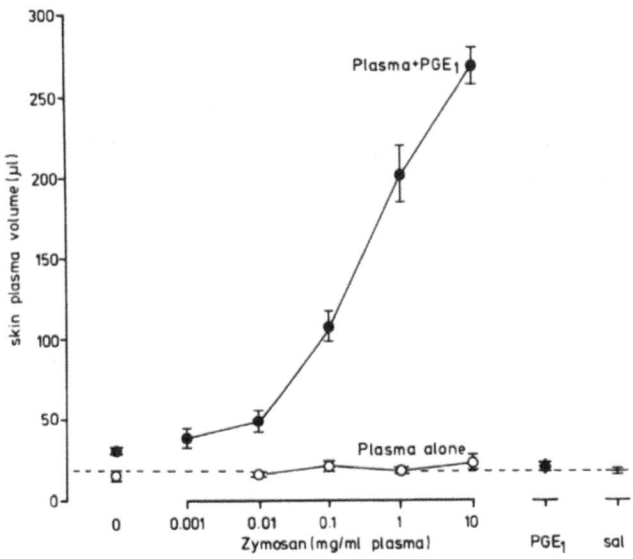

FIGURE 2. Oedema induced in rabbit skin by intradermal injections
of zymosan-activated plasma.   Plasma was incubated (37°C for 30 min)
with zymosan at the concentrations shown.   The zymosan was then
removed by centrifugation and the plasma injected into skin in
0.1 ml volumes with and without PGE_1 (3×10^{-10}mol/0.1ml).
Results are shown as means $\pm$ s.e.mean (n=6).

5. A LINK BETWEEN POLYMORPHONUCLEAR NEUTROPHILS AND INCREASED
MICROVASCULAR PERMEABILITY

Two lines of evidence indicated that C5a did not owe its activity on
the microvasculature to a release of histamine from mast cells.   Firstly,
responses to C5a, like those to intradermally-injected zymosan, were not
abolished by anti-histamines (4).   Secondly, carboxyl terminal arginine is
necessary for histamine release in some species and removal of this group
(leaving C5a des Arg) did not abolish activity; (this has now been
demonstrated in human plasma (6)).   Initially, our interpretation of these
findings was that C5a was able to act directly on microvessels to cause
leakage.   However, several clues pointed to a connection between activities
on PMN neutrophils observed *in vitro* and microvascular responses *in vivo*.

154

Firstly, both C5a and C5a des Arg are active as chemotactic agents *in vitro*. Secondly, we found that other substances with chemotactic activity, N-formyl-methionyl-leucyl-phenylalanine and leukotriene B_4, were also able to induce oedema in skin when the substances were mixed with a vasodilator prostaglandin (3). Thirdly, there was a latent period before leakage was detectable after intradermal injection of C5a + PGE_2 and this latent period was not observed when using bradykinin + PGE_2 or histamine + PGE_2 (3). Figure 3 shows the result of such an experiment.

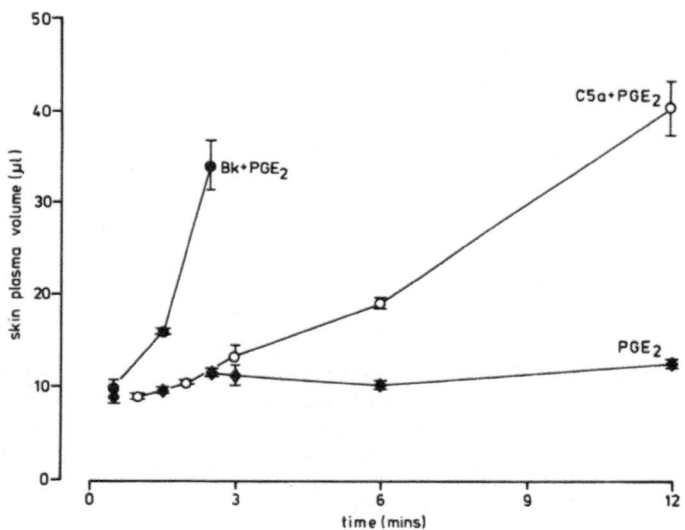

FIGURE 3. A comparison of the onset time of leakage induced by intradermal injections of C5a + PGE_2 and bradykinin + PGE_2; PGE_2 serves as control. Doses/0.1 ml were C5a 1.5×10^{-11} mol, bradykinin 5×10^{-10} mol, PGE_2 3×10^{-10} mol. The injections were given at different times (shown on the abscissa) before killing the rabbit. Note the latent period before responses to C5a + PGE_2 are apparent. Results are shown as means $\pm$ s.e.mean (n=4).

Finally, no responses to C5a + PGE_2 could be obtained in rabbits depleted of circulating PMN neutrophils whereas responses to bradykinin + PGE_2 and histamine + PGE_2 were unaffected (3). An example of such an experiment is shown in Fig.4.

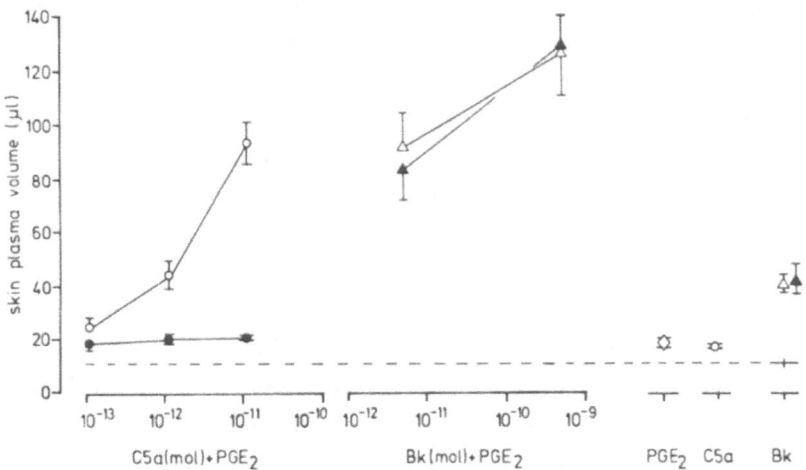

FIGURE 4. Oedema induced in rabbit skin by C5a + PGE_2 and bradykinin + PGE_2: the effect of depletion of PMN neutrophils. Responses in normal animals (n = 6-16) are shown as open symbols. Responses in depleted animals (n = 6-16) are shown as closed symbols. Rabbits were depleted of circulating PMN neutrophils using single intravenous injections of 1.75 mg nitrogen mustard/kg and tested 4 days later.

These results support the hypothesis (3,6) that C5a injected, or generated, extravascularly triggers a very rapid interaction between circulating PMN neutrophils and venular endothelial cells and that this interaction results in an increase in permeability to macromolecules.

Whether increased permeability results from the passage of the leukocyte out of the vessel between endothelial cells, from the release of a secretory product by the leukocyte, or from a direct cell-cell interaction, remains to be established.

6. CONCLUSION

Protein leakage from the microvascular bed has been generally regarded as a consequence of injury to the blood vessel wall. It has been proposed, for example, that vessel walls can be injured by: complement mediated lytic processes; enzymes released from leukocytes during phagocytosis; and superoxide released during phacocytosis. Similarly, various chemical mediators are often said to cause vessel wall injury. This concept has been reinforced by recent work on the intravascular generation of C5a which has been correlated with microvascular injury in the lung.

Whilst inflammation undoubtedly does result in injured vessels in some circumstances, the question should be asked: is protein leakage merely a disagreeable byproduct of the defence process? Alternatively, taking a specific case in the context of the results described here: have mechanisms evolved to recognise byproducts of complement activation, such as C5a, in order to put into effect a necessary component of the defence process? When complement activation is regarded as essentially a local extravascular event, such a concept of 'functional oedema' becomes plausible. In spite of the fact that C5a was originally described as an activity generated intravascularly, this site may be of less importance in nature. Certainly, many of the descriptions of intravascular generation of the substance are a consequence of a factitious interference with the circulation.

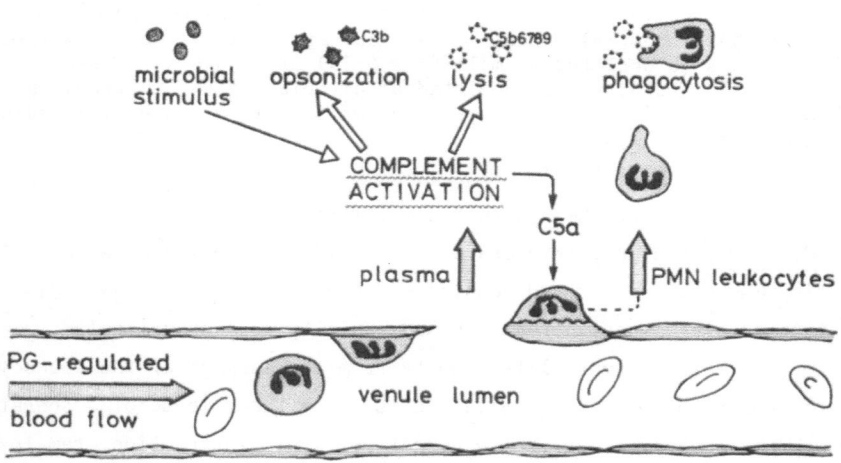

FIGURE 5. The microvascular response to C5a - a proposed system for controlling the supply of complement and phagocytes to an infected tissue.

Figure 5 shows the proposed sequence of events following the injection of tissue with microbes.   Activation of the complement sequence can begin immediately in extracellular tissue fluid.   This results in opsonization (coating of microbes with C3b), lysis (by the 'attack sequence' C5b6789), followed by phagocytosis of opsonized particles by PMN neutrophils.   These processes would very quickly deplete complement available locally if a system were not available to supply more from blood plasma.   Since the mechanisms which exist to eliminate microbes involve their pretreatment by the complement system before phagocytosis, this may explain why the phagocytes are involved with the supply of complement to the tissue from the blood.   This may or may not be the reason, but nevertheless a byproduct of complement activation, C5a, appears to control the accumulation of PMN leukocytes and these cells in turn (by some unknown mechanism) control the leakage of plasma components into the tissue.

An experimental analysis of this working hypothesis and a determination of the relevance of mechanisms of this type to more complex inflammatory reactions may prove fruitful in the future.

I thank my colleagues Drs. Peter Jose, Caroline Wedmore and Michael Forrest for allowing me to refer to work carried out in collaboration. Much of this work was financed by the Medical Research Council, U.K.

REFERENCES

1.   Williams, T.J. & Morley, J. (1973).   Prostaglandins as potentiators of increased vascular permeability in inflammation.   Nature, $\underline{246}$, 215-217.
2.   Williams, T.J. & Peck, M.J.   (1977). Role of prostaglandin-mediated vasodilatation in inflammation.   Nature, $\underline{270}$, 530-532.
3.   Wedmore, C.V. & Williams, T.J.   (1981)   Control of vascular permeability by polymorphonuclear leukocytes in inflammation. Nature, $\underline{289}$, 646-650.
4.   Williams, T.J. & Jose, P.J.   (1981)   Mediation of increased vascular permeability after complement activation: histamine-independent action of rabbit C5a.   J.exp.Med., $\underline{153}$, 135-153.
5.   Williams, T.J.   (1979)   Prostaglandin E_2, prostaglandin I_2 and the vascular changes in inflammation.   Br.J.Pharmac., $\underline{65}$, 517-524.
6.   Jose, P.J., Forrest, M.J. & Williams, T.J.   (1981)   Human C5a des Arg increases vascular permeability.   J.Immunol., (in press)

LEUCOCYTE LOCOMOTION ON TWO-DIMENSIONAL SURFACES AND
IN THREE-DIMENSIONAL MATRICES

P. C. WILKINSON, WENDY S. HASTON AND J. M. SHIELDS

1. INTRODUCTION

We wish to discuss here an important determinant of leucocyte
locomotion that has not received much consideration, namely the
structure and shape of the substratum   on which, or within
which, the cell moves. Recent progress in the study of leucocyte
locomotion has been centred not so much on the cells' physical environment as on the biochemical control of locomotion, and especially
on the biochemistry of chemotaxis. Chemotaxis is almost certainly
the major mechanism by which leucocytes accumulate in acute inflammatory sites. However, the assay systems we use to study it in vitro
do not do justice to the complexity of the tissues through which leucocytes must move to reach those inflammatory sites in vivo. Most
tissues of the body are three-dimensional and, in connective tissue,
sheets of collagen fibrils frequently show alignment. Thus neither
the flat protein-coated glass coverslips used for filming assays nor
the porous but unaligned meshwork of the micropore filters used in
many chemotactic assays necessarily provide an environment similar
to that met by cells in the body. In vivo, leucocytes must be able
to move both in three dimensional meshworks, such as connective
tissue, and on planar surfaces such as the serous lining of body
cavities. We know that on planar surfaces locomotion is dependent
on adhesion, and the cells must grip the surface to pull themselves
forward. It is less obvious that cells need to adhere to 3-D lattices.
They may instead move by using these as climbing frames, gaining
purchase from non-adhesive contacts in the lattice. These ideas will

be explored below. We wish to consider in turn three aspects of
the influence of the substratum on leucocyte locomotion: (a) the
ability of leucocytes to detect solid-phase gradients, i.e. chemotactic
molecules bound to glass coverslips to form a stable gradient;
(b) the effect of the shape of the substratum and the possibility that
leucocyte locomotion is guided by the contours of the surfaces the
cells move on. These were studied using neutrophil leucocytes which
are known to adhere well; (c) the special problem of locomotion of
lymphocytes which adhere very poorly to most protein-coated surfaces,
and mechanisms by which these non-adherent cells are nevertheless
able to move actively through tissues.

2. NEUTROPHIL CHEMOTAXIS ON SURFACE-BOUND GRADIENTS

The first problem we wish to discuss is the role of the substratum
in chemotaxis of neutrophil leucocytes. Chemotactic factors, especially proteins, bind appreciably to surfaces, so that chemotactic gradients may be formed, not only in free solution, but also on the surfaces
along which cells move. Do leucocytes respond to these gradients
of solid-phase attractants or only to fluid-phase gradients or to both?
The cell membrane receptors of leucocytes crawling over a chemo-
tactic-factor-coated substratum are likely to bind sequentially to substratum-bound ligands as the cell moves forward in a manner remin-
iscent of the 'zipper' mechanism by which phagocytosis proceeds by
sequential attachment of receptor sites on the plasma membrane of
advancing pseudopods to ligands distributed evenly around the circumference of the particle being ingested (1, 2). We asked ourselves
whether chemotaxis could likewise proceed by sequential attachment
of cell-surface receptors on the advancing lamellipodium to ligands
bound to the substratum. To do this, we had to make solid-phase
gradients of chemotactic factors in the absence of the same factor
in free solution. Preliminary evidence that neutrophils could respond
to substratum-bound chemotactic factors in the absence of fluid-phase
attractant came from Dierich et al. (3) who exposed micropore filters

to the chemotactic factor, casein, then washed away all of the protein
except that which had bound to the filter. Cells placed on the top
surface of such filters moved as far into the filter in response to the
filter-bound casein as they did in a control experiment in which casein
was present in the fluid phase. These experiments showed that a
surface-bound attractant could stimulate neutrophil locomotion, but
not that the locomotion was chemotactic. We used two types of assay
to test this. In the first, we used the filter assay and set up a
'checkerboard' of solid-phase casein gradients on a series of filters.
We then placed neutrophils on top of these filters and allowed them
to migrate in in the usual way. Neutrophils migrated further into the
filters in response to positive filter-bound gradients than to negative
filter-bound gradients (4), a result that was consistent with a chemotactic response. We later obtained stronger evidence for chemotaxis
on substratum-bound gradients using a visual assay (5). A gradient
of a chemotactic protein (casein or denatured human serum albumin)
was formed along the surface of a glass coverslip using the orientation
chamber described by Zigmond (6). The coverslip was washed to
remove fluid-phase protein but leaving the gradient of solid-phase protein in situ. Neutrophils were then allowed to settle on such coverslips and their locomotion was filmed. These cells showed a significant directional bias of locomotion up-gradient from low concentrations
towards high concentrations of the substratum-bound proteins (Table 1).
The suggestion that neutrophils detect substratum-bound chemotactic
factors is also supported by studies using gradients of the chemotactic
factor, C5a bound to micropore filters (7). In the presence of serum
albumin, human neutrophils migrated into the filters in response to
the filter-bound C5a-gradient. It therefore seems clear that neutrophils do detect and move up substratum-bound gradients of chemotactic
factors, probably using a mechanism that resembles the 'zippering'
process. It is less obvious that detection of solid-phase gradients is
the only mechanism by which neutrophils migrate towards chemotactic

Table 1. Displacement of human neutrophils on substratum-bound gradients of chemotactic proteins.

	No. of cells	Mean speed (μm/min)	Mean displacement towards gradient source (μm/min $\pm$ S.E.M.)	Mean displacement parallel to gradient source (μm/min $\pm$ S.E.M.)
Casein gradient (original conc^n. 0-1mg/ml)	25	15.3	5.3$\pm$1.4. p.001	0.98$\pm$1.7. p$\rangle$0.1
Alkali-denatured HSA gradient (original conc^n. 0-8mg/ml	42	7.6	2.2$\pm$0.5. p.0001	0.66$\pm$0.6. p$\rangle$0.1

sources, or the most important one. It is equally possible that fluid-phase chemotactic molecules, diffusing in a gradient, can bind to cell surface receptors and stimulate orientation of the cells in the gradient even under conditions where the chemotactic molecules remain unbound to the substratum, as suggested by observations of chemotactic-factor-induced polarization of leucocytes in suspension (8). Small chemotactic formyl-peptides activate neutrophils whether or not the cells are attached to a surface, though for locomotion to these peptides, a protein-coated surface is essential, possibly because such surfaces promote the right kind of adhesion to allow locomotion. At present, we feel that the 'zippering' mechanism is one way, but not the only way, for leucocytes to detect and move up chemotactic gradients.

3. CONTACT GUIDANCE

By contact guidance we mean a directionality of cellular orientation or locomotion determined by the physical structure or shape of the substratum. Cells show a preference for movement in the axis of alignment of an aligned tissue over other axes. Their locomotion is bidirectional, up and down the axis, unlike chemotaxis which is unidirectional. Cells have been known for many years to align along fibrin strands or collagen fibrils (9). There have been several careful recent studies of guidance using fibroblasts (10-12). Strangely however, the possibility that leucocytes show guidance has not been explored.

Our first study (Wilkinson, Shields and Haston, in preparation) was of the locomotion of human blood neutrophils on a very familiar surface, namely that of a grooved glass Neubauer counting chamber. The neutrophils were suspended in 20 percent normal serum, so they were moving on protein-coated glass. They showed a striking preference for movement along the grooves of the counting grid rather than on plane glass, and many of the cells, which were on plane glass at the beginning of filming, joined grooves, so that after 15 minutes almost all cells were moving on grooves.

We next turned to the use of more physiological surfaces, namely aligned fibrous gels of collagen or of fibrin. Gelation of collagen was achieved by manipulation of the pH and ionic strength of collagen maintained in solution in acetic acid. Once the collagen was restored to physiological pH and ionic strength, it formed a gel. Fibrin gels were formed by adding thrombin to fibrinogen. The gels were aligned by putting tension on them. There are several ways to do this, i.e. gentle traction with filter papers on both ends of the gel, or forming the gel on a sloping surface, or stroking in one direction with a fine paintbrush as the gel forms. Neutrophils were incorporated into the forming gel and their movement in the aligned gel was filmed. There was an unequivocal preference for locomotion in or near the axis of alignment of the gel fibres over locomotion across the axis of alignment (Table 2). These cells were moving within a three-dimensional fibrous matrix. When the gels were dried down to form a flat surface of aligned fibres, the cells no longer showed contact guidance. This observation is similar to that of Dunn and Ebendal (11) who observed fibroblast orientation in the axis of alignment of 3-D collagen gels but not after the gels had been dried. Dunn (13) has suggested some possible mechanisms for guidance, one being that the shape of moving cells is subject to less distortion when the cells are polarized along

Table 2. Angles made by segments* of paths of 26 neutrophils to axis of alignment of a collagen gel.

Number of segments at angle between $0°$ and $29°$	223	χ^2 test shows significant differ-
Number of segments at angle between $30°$ and $59°$	151	ence between all three
Number of segments at angle between $60°$ and $90°$	90	
Total	464	

*Each segment is the straight-line distance travelled by a cell during 40 seconds.

the fibres than when polarized across them, so that pull might be exerted more efficiently by microfilaments in the former than in the latter cells. Another possible mechanism follows from the fact that the aligned fibres are elastic and under tension. When a cell pulls at right angles to such a fibre, it distorts it like a plucked string, and much of the purchase necessary for locomotion is lost, whereas when a cell pulls along the axis of alignment of the fibre, the fibre is less distorted, and most of the traction is instead used in pulling the cell forward. Both possibilities would account for guidance responses in hydrated 3-D gels aligned under tension, and the loss of guidance on dried, aligned gels which are no longer under tension. These mechanisms remain to be explored in leucocytes. The fact that leucocytes show guidance responses must be taken into account in considering inflammatory responses in vivo since the tissues through which the cells move frequently show alignment or more complex forms of patterning. Chemotactic responses may be more efficient when cells are moving along aligned tissues than across them.

4. NECESSITY FOR 3-D SUBSTRATA FOR LOCOMOTION OF LYMPHOCYTES

Both reactions discussed above depend on close adhesion of neutrophil leucocytes to a substratum. The study of lymphocyte locomotion and of chemotactic reactions in lymphocytes presents special problems since lymphocytes are well-known to be poorly adhesive to most commonly-used surfaces; in fact this property is often used

in methods for their purification from other, adhesive, cell-types.
Nevertheless, lymphocytes are actively motile both in vitro and in
vivo and motility is essential to their recirculation through lymphoid
tissue and their recruitment into inflammatory sites (14).   A number
of groups including our own have now shown chemotactic reactions in
lymphocytes using the filter assay (14), but we have failed repeatedly
to demonstrate the same reactions by filming lymphocytes moving on
plane substrata.   When lymphocytes are placed in contact with a variety of cell-types in tissue culture, e.g. lymph node reticular cells or
fibroblasts, they move poorly on the cell-free substratum, but show
rapid movement while underlapping the reticular cells or fibroblasts
(15-17).   These observations raise the possibility that the space between the tissue cell and the substratum provides a three-dimensional
environment suitable for lymphocyte movement, whereas their grip on
a plane surface is insufficient to give the traction necessary for movement.   Likewise the lattice of a filter, but not a plane glass surface,
allows the lymphocytes to respond to chemotactic factors.   Having
failed to obtain substantial lymphocyte attachment to, or locomotion
on, plane surfaces coated with a variety of proteins including fibronectin, casein and whole serum, we decided to study their behaviour
within the matrix of hydrated 3-D collagen gels (non-aligned), compared
to dried collagen (Haston, Shields and Wilkinson, submitted for publication).   These experiments were performed using lymphocytes from
the peripheral lymph nodes of unprimed mice.   We found that lymphocytes placed on the surface of a 3-D collagen gel attached well to
the gel and were able to penetrate into, and move actively within,
its matrix (Table 3).   When the gel was dried down, lymphocytes no
longer attached to it or moved on it.   When such dried gels were re-
hydrated, lymphocytes were again able to attach to and penetrate the
gel.   These experiments support the idea that a 3-D matrix is necessary for locomotion.   A possible reason why this might be so is
suggested by filming studies.   Moving lymphocytes within gels extend

Table 3. Lymphocyte attachment to hydrated (3-D) and dried (2-D) collagen gels

Treatment of coverslips	No. of cells attached per field (Mean of 15 fields $\pm$ S.D.)
Hydrated collagen gel	57 ± 6
Dried collagen coat	16 ± 3
Collagen dried and rehydrated	90 ± 11

pseudopods which they appear to be able to protrude into gaps in the lattice and which then expand on the opposite side of the gap. In this way, the cells seemed able to gain purchase, either to push themselves away from the gap, or for the cell body to follow the pseudopod through the gap. This form of locomotion would not require any close adhesive contact between the lymphocyte and the collagen, since the cell is really simply using the collagen as a climbing frame. We tested the idea that pseudopod insertion was important by studying lymphocyte attachment to protein-coated cellulose ester filters of various poresizes. Lymphocytes should only be able to attach to filters with pores big enough for the cell to insert a pseudopod and thus anchor itself. In fact, in a distraction assay, lymphocytes showed good attachment to filters of 3.0 and 8.0μm poresizes, but not to those of the same material but of 0.22 or 0.45μm poresizes. The latter probably do not permit insertion of a sizeable pseudopod. We therefore suggest that lymphocyte locomotion proceeds by an adhesion-independent mechanism that requires that the cell gain contacts by pseudopod insertion into gaps or cavities in three-dimensional environments such as fibrous matrices, or possibly into the spaces between apposed surfaces of tissue cells.

5. CONCLUSIONS

Our conclusions from these studies are as follows.

(a) Neutrophils move well by making adhesive contacts with plane substrata. They are able to detect solid-phase gradients of chemotactic factors bound to such substrata.

(b) In aligned 3-D matrices, neutrophils show contact guidance with a preference for locomotion in the axis of alignment.

(c) Lymphocytes are non-adhesive cells and move poorly on plane substrata. However they move efficiently in 3-D matrices, gaining support by protrusion of pseudopods into gaps in the matrix, a mechanism that does not require close adhesion.

This work was supported by the Medical Research Council.

REFERENCES

1. Griffin FM, Griffin JA, Leider JE and Silverstein SC, 1975. J. exp. Med. 142 1263-1282.
2. Griffin FM, Griffin JA and Silverstein SC, 1976. J. exp. Med. 144 788-809.
3. Dierich MP, Wilhelmi D and Till G, 1977. Nature 270 351-352.
4. Wilkinson PC and Allan RB 1978. Exp. Cell Res. 117 403-412.
5. Wilkinson PC and Bradley GR 1981. Immunology 42 637-648.
6. Zigmond SH 1977. J. Cell Biol. 75 606-616.
7. Webster RO, Zanolari B and Henson PM 1980. Exp. Cell Res. 129 55-62.
8. Cianciolo GJ and Snyderman R 1981. J. Clin. Invest. 67 60-68.
9. Weiss P. 1959. Rev. Mod. Phys. 31 11-20.
10. Dunn GA and Heath JP 1976. Exp. Cell Res. 101 1-14.
11. Dunn GA and Ebendal T 1978. Exp. Cell Res. 111 475-479.
12. O'Hara PT and Buck RC, 1979. Exp. Cell Res. 121 235-249.
13. Dunn GA 1981 in Biology of the Chemotactic Response, ed. JM Lackie and PC Wilkinson, Cambridge University Press, Cambridge, in press.
14. Parrott DMV and Wilkinson PC 1981. Prog. Allergy. 28, 193-284.
15. Ponten J 1975 in Cancer, Vol. 4 ed. FF Becker, pp 55-100, Plenum, New York.
16. Haston WS 1979. Cell. Immunol. 45 74-84.
17. Chang TW, Celis E, Eisen HN and Solomon F 1979. Proc. Nat. Acad. Sci. U.S.A. 76 2917-2921.

CELL - SURFACE INTERACTIONS: EFFECTS ON VASCULAR PERMEABILITY
AND ON WBC LOCOMOTION (COMMENTARY)

R. R. MACGREGOR

LEUCOCYTE LOCOMOTION ON TWO-DIMENSIONAL SURFACES AND IN THREE-
DIMENSIONAL MATRICES

The PMN's ability to respond to a solid-phase gradient was
examined by Dr Wilkinson and co-workers by binding chemotactic
factors to micropore filters and glass coverslips and then ob-
serving PMN's movements in the presence of these gradients. Results supported the thesis that PMNs can recognize a solid-phase
gradient of a chemotactic factor and move up the gradient by
fastening sequentially to fixed molecules of chemotactic factor,
"zippering" the membrane to the surface via its chemotactic
factor receptors. This model does not explain how the cell
recognizes an increasing concentration, nor how it "unzippers"
its membrane on the trailing edge of the gradient. Moreover, it
is not clear that the solid-phase gradient remains totally in the
solid phase; when the fluid suspension of PMNs is added, some
fluid-phase gradient may be re-established by elution of chemotactic factor from the solid phase.

In pointing out the importance of contact guidance, Dr Wilkinson makes an important contribution to our understanding of in
vivo chemotaxis. Using three-dimensional gel matrices of collagen
or fibrin, whose fibres had been aligned by tension applied to
the gel, they showed that PMNs moved preferentially along the
axis of alignment of the fibers. This finding is significant to
the in vivo situation, in which most connective tissue contains
collagen fibres which are aligned. A complicating factor may be
that oedema and necrosis associated with inflammation may have
an unpredictable effect on a tissue's fibre alignment.

168

Finally, Dr Wilkinson sheds light on the puzzle of why lymphocytes move poorly along planes, but well in 3-dimensional
matrices. Noting that lymphocytes do not adhere well to surfaces
and thus would have difficulty pulling themselves along, he
theorizes that they climb a matrix like a ladder. A pseudopod is
thrust through a small hole and then expanded until it wedges,
offering "purchase" for the cell then to pull itself forward. His
demonstration that lymphocytes will adhere to filters of large
pore size but not to those with very small pores (0.22 or 0.45 µm)
is suggestive. A useful confirming experiment would be to fix the
cells on these filters and to demonstrate on cross-section microscopy of the filter that the cells are, or are not, inserting
pseudopodia into the pores to gain "footholds".

INCREASED VASCULAR PERMEABILITY FOLLOWING INTERACTION BETWEEN
NUCLEAR NEUTROPHILS AND VASCULAR ENDOTHELIAL CELLS

Dr Williams and his colleagues have demonstrated that the
development of oedema during inflammation requires the syner-
gistic action of two mediators, one which causes vasodilatation
and one resulting in increased vascular permeability. Using
prostaglandin E_1 as the vasodilator and zymosan-activated serum
(containing C5a) as the permeability factor, they showed that
neither produced oedema alone, but that their combined use led
to a significant plasma leakage. An elegant paper in the 1981
Journal of Experimental Medicine (4) offers convincing evidence
that the permeability factor is C5a. If so, one would predict
that serum treatment by endotoxin or by antigen-antibody complex
would have the same effect as zymosan.

The evidence that C5a exerts ist permeability-inducing effect
through its action on PMNs is indirect but suggestive. The fact
that PMN-depleted rabbits fail to develop oedema in response to
C5a and PGE_2 is the most convincing. The mechanism by which PMNs
increase permeability is unknown, but Dr Williams suggests three
possibilities: 1. As a result of their diapedesis,2. Secretion of
a permeability-inducing factor by PMNs, 3. Direct PMN action on

the endothelial cell. A recent paper by Dale and co-workers
(J. Clin. Invest. 1981, 67: 584) has demonstrated that PMNs
can pass through intercellular junctions of endothelial monolayers without allowing protein passage, a finding which makes
mechanism number 1 unlikely to lead to significant oedema. PMNs
are rich in lysosomal enzymes, and can secrete them into the
environment when suitably stimulated. The injection of these
enzymes into Dr Williams experimental model might offer data to
support mechanism number 2. However, transmission electron
microscopy of PMNs adhering to and moving between endothelial
cells during inflammation (Q.J. Exper. Physiol. 1960, 45: 343)
does not show degranulation or evidence of secretory activity.
Mechanism number 3, direct damage of endothelial cells by PMNs
does have some supportive evidence. C5a increases PMN adherence
to endothelial cells (and to other surfaces), and this can cause
protein leakage in the pulmonary vasculature (N. Engl. J. Med.
1977, 296: 769). This damage could lead to widening of intercellular spaces, with subsequent protein leakage. But again,
transmission electron microscopy does not show morphologic
changes in the cells of endothelium being traversed by PMNs
during inflammation.

Dr Williams reminds us that the vascular leak of plasma
supplies plasma proteins, many of which are involved in host
defence mechanims such as the complement system, to the extravascular sites where they can be utilized to the benefit of the
host.